The Exercise Hack

How to form a lasting exercise habit and finally be in the best shape of your life

Caitlyn Tanner, Pharm.D

The Exercise Hack

How to form a lasting exercise habit and finally be in the best shape of your life

By Caitlyn Tanner, Pharm.D.

ISBN:979-8-9907218-0-7

Table of Contents

To my family and friends.
Thank you for believing in me, especially
when I didn't even believe in myself.

Disclaimer

The material in this book is intended to appeal to a broad audience, so it includes topics in a general sense. No two human beings are exactly alike; even identical twins have unique fingerprints. Please keep this in mind while consuming this material. I am a licensed healthcare professional but I am not *your* healthcare professional. It is important to consult a specialist regarding your unique situation before taking general health and wellness advice.

Further, the concepts discussed are intentionally simplified to make them more easily digestible for people who are new to regular exercise or struggling to adopt an exercise habit. While fitness and exercise are both studied and practiced with attention to their many microscopic details, they are not covered here with much granularity.

Finally, the material in this book was not created using artificial intelligence, but my own human mind. The utility of robots is growing at an unprecedented rate, but the content

Disclaimer

contained herein is reflective of my own authentic human knowledge, work, and experience peppered with my ridiculous sense of humor. I researched the referenced scientific data and information myself. You can review the references for this book's content at the end of the printed and electronic versions and on the website, www.theexercisehack.com.

Introduction

Who writes a book about exercise?

It would be cool and exciting if I could start this book by tooting my own horn and telling you that I am an award-winning heart surgeon. Or that I've finished seven ironman triathlons and stood on the podium every time. Or that I am a personal trainer for a famous Olympic athlete. But I'm not going to do that. Because none of that is true.

Don't get me wrong; I've done some noteworthy and interesting things in my life, but I'm just a regular person. I'm not an elite athlete, a fitness model, or a vegan yogi who eats quinoa and makes spinach smoothies every Sunday. I'm a middle-aged mother of two who figured out how to start an exercise routine and keep it going until I got six-pack abs. I've cycled through all of the yo-yo dieting and the As Seen on TV fitness devices, and I've been overweight and out of shape several times in my life. In 2006, I was so "fluffy," you could have easily mistaken me for the Michelin Man. A number of years and two kids later, when I finally got into the shape that I had always wanted to be in, complete strangers started approaching me and asking how I got so fit. It was awkward at first, especially when I was at the grocery store and a man with prosthetic legs told me I had nice, muscular legs. I had been so focused on my fitness goals that I hadn't realized anyone else noticed. After at least a dozen of these types of encounters, I figured that maybe I had enough experience to dole out some advice. After all, people *were* asking.

I'm also a pharmacist, so I have a little background in health sciences. And I've spent my entire adult life trying to figure out the easiest way *not* to have to take all the medications I've been peddling. You know, the ones for diabetes, high cholesterol, high blood pressure, heart disease, and other diseases. Many of the diseases these medications treat are strongly linked to obesity. Obesity is an epidemic of such large proportions (pun intended) that it spans much of the globe. The World Health Organization (WHO) is actually now calling it "globesity." It's no newsflash that what most ails us in Western society can be simply corrected with a proper diet and exercise. We've had this information for years, yet we still can't seem to put the necessary lifestyle changes in motion to correct our society's obesity epidemic and its associated effects. Working in healthcare for over twenty years, I've given millions of people advice on their health. And the one piece of advice that seems to be the absolute hardest for most people to follow is "get more exercise" (second maybe to "eat a better diet" and "stop smoking"). Healthcare work put me in the business of helping people. I wrote this book because I want the information contained herein to help people more than pill pushing does. As the idiom goes, an ounce of prevention is worth a pound of cure.

Why not write about health in general? Or exercise and diet together?

I'm guessing this isn't the first book you've read about getting healthy. If it is, then I'm honored that you've chosen this one. There are hundreds of so-called "get healthy" books out there. I know because I've read them myself. They tell you a wide variety of things you should be doing, like eating more vegetables, getting at least eight hours of sleep, drinking at least eight glasses of water, meditating, not smoking or drinking alcohol, and on and on. And when you've finished reading them, you've realized you might be even more unhealthy than you originally thought and you're *very* overwhelmed with all the changes you need to make. My guess is that you tried some or all of the recommendations, but eventually decided that it's all too much and too hard, and you ended up throwing in the towel and finding yourself back at square one.

It's true—doing all of these things will definitely make you healthier—but is it realistic to expect someone to make *all* these changes to their habits and lifestyle at once? In my experience, it's not only unrealistic, but it sets people up for failure and disappointment. The hard truth about changing your habits to be healthier is that the changes need to be *permanent*. Not just for seventy-five days or until you lose the weight but for the rest of your life. And the best way to make positive changes that last for the rest of your life is to focus (I mean *really* focus) on one change at a time until you consider the change permanent. In this book, we're going to focus on changing your exercise habits (or lack thereof) for the rest of your life.

For whom is this book written?

So not to waste anyone's time, this book might not benefit the person who already has their fitness routine completely dialed in. If you have a fitness routine that has worked for you for the last five to ten years and you don't feel the need to take it to the next level, this book might not be what you are looking for.

However, this book might help you if any of the following conditions sound familiar:

1. A healthcare worker has told you to start exercising.

2. You want and/or need to lose weight with exercise.

3. You live a sedentary life and want to live healthier by moving more.

4. You like exercise, but you lack motivation to do it on a regular basis.

5. You think exercise was invented by Satan himself, but you know you should still be doing it.

6. You want to look better naked, but an exercise routine seems unattainable.

7. You made a New Year's resolution to start exercising regularly, and you quit by St. Patrick's Day.

If you've seen any of these movies before, and you're not living happily ever after as a result, then follow me through the rest of this book so we can rewrite the endings.

Chapter 1

Where Are We and How Did We Get Here?

Health is not valued till sickness comes.
—*Thomas Fuller*

Let's face it: Americans are fat. (No, I'm not calling you fat; I'm calling *us* fat). According to the Centers for Disease Control and Prevention (CDC), in the past twenty years (from 2000 to 2020), the prevalence of obesity went from 30.5 percent to almost 42.0 percent with severe obesity increasing from 4.7 percent to 9.2 percent. This means that two of every five Americans are considered obese and one in ten are severely obese. To make matters worse, as of the date this book was written, one in five American children aged two to nineteen are also obese. The consequences of obesity are plentiful. It is responsible for increasing a person's risk of heart disease, type 2 diabetes, breathing problems, joint problems, gallbladder disease, strokes, anxiety, depression, certain types of cancer and premature death. (Wow, that sounded like the side effects list from a pharmaceutical TV ad).

How did this happen!?

If you look at old photos, magazines, TV shows, and movies from decades past, you'll notice that we weren't always this fat. I recently showed my kids the classic 1986 movie *Stand By Me*. In this movie, Jerry O'Connell plays "the fat kid" of a group of four friends. When he referred to himself as "the fat kid" in the movie, my nine-year-old son turned to me with confusion and said, "he isn't even fat though." And he was right. By today's standards, we would hesitate to say that Jerry O'Connell's character is overweight at all, no less obese. In 1970, only 15 percent of adults and 5 percent of children aged two to nineteen in the US were considered obese. So in just fifty years, the number of obese American adults has more than doubled, and for children, it has nearly quadrupled! How did this happen? And why does it only seem to be getting worse? To answer the first question, we have to look at what has changed between then and now.

Multiple studies have suggested that the increase in obesity rates from the 1970s to the 2020s are directly correlated with an increase in sugar consumption. But it's not just sugar calories we've increased in our diets over that time span. It's *all* calories. Portion sizes have dramatically increased as well as how often we eat out. High-calorie, highly addictive foods have become more affordable, widely available, and heavily advertised. Our food has become much more processed than it once was. If you have children, think back to when you were a child. How is your own child's diet different from the one your parents offered you? If you have the ability, and you'd like to make this activity even more interesting, ask your parents what their diets looked like when they were children. The availability and choice of poor quality foods has spiraled out of control with every subsequent generation. But it isn't just our dietary changes to blame for fattening us up over the past half century.

Enter, technology. The year 1981 gave birth to the first IBM personal computer (PC) and with it, a rise in screen time. If the PC wasn't enough to distract you from the already popular television screen, you could also plug in your new video game console for even more hours of fun. Since the 1980s, the video gaming industry has continued to grow exponentially. We can also give credit to the 1980s for the improvements in cellular technology. Cell phones were too expensive then for most people, but by the 1990s, they were increasingly more affordable and practical. The 1990s saw a sharp rise in internet usage as well. And as the 2000s approached, cell phones and other mobile computer devices such as laptops, tablets, and handheld computers were commonplace.

Social media entered the scene (or should I say screen?) in 2004 and has also grown exponentially since its inception. While many of these technological advances have improved our quality of life, as technology has grown, so have our midsections. Every year since the 1980s, we have spent more and more time staring at screens and sitting on our backsides. According to 2022 data from DataReportal, the average American spends seven hours looking at a screen every day. Screen time has become an enormous part of our work, pleasure, and communication. But screen time is sedentary time. This sedentary way of life crept in slowly and quietly over decades. We are all victims to it. Those screens are captivating and they suck us all into their brightly lit vortex. I'm staring into one now as I write this book.

The sedentary lifestyle has taken over

So let's talk about the evolution of technology in relation to our employment. As technology has improved, the use of screens has become more and more relevant to our professional productivity. The American Heart Association (AHA) says that sedentary jobs have increased by 83 percent since 1950. Physically active jobs now make up less than 20 percent of the US workforce, down from roughly half of jobs in 1960. Recent studies estimate the average American adult sits between eight and eleven hours per day. We wake up in the morning, sit to eat breakfast, sit in a car, bus, or train for our commute to work, sit in front of a desk for at least eight hours, sit for the commute home, sit down at the dinner table, sit on the couch, then lay down to sleep, and do the same thing the next day. We basically live in captivity, rotating through our cages. At my last corporate job, I spent more than forty hours per week confined to a cage although most people call them cubicles.

If a sharp rise in sitting and screen time weren't bad enough, over time we've capitalized on making almost everything in our daily lives more convenient. We hire out laborious household tasks such as trimming the yard, washing windows, and shampooing the carpets. Instead of shopping for our own groceries, pushing a shopping cart through each isle of a store, we can order online with delivery to our doorstep. We can use a delivery service to purchase a meal that someone else prepared for us. We can order almost anything our hearts desire on the internet for home delivery without even getting out of our armchairs. What an amazing time to be alive—and to put almost no physical effort into anything.

The consequences are grim

Most Americans have likely heard more than once that the most common cause of obesity is poor diet and lack of exercise. Simply put, obesity is augmented by having too much energy input (e.g., food) and not enough energy output (e.g., physical activity). But what if you can maintain a healthy diet and weight without much exercise or physical movement? Well, independent of the risk for obesity or actual obesity itself, physical inactivity still increases a person's risk for heart disease, stroke, metabolic syndrome, type 2 diabetes, certain types of cancers, osteoporosis, falls, anxiety, depression, and premature death. So if you live a sedentary lifestyle, and you've successfully dodged the associated obesity, your health risks still look a lot like the ones you would have if you were obese. Further, even if your weight remains in an overweight or obese category, you can greatly reduce the risks associated with carrying excess weight by getting regular exercise.

Despite the common knowledge that exercise is necessary to live a long, healthful life, the CDC reported in 2022 that roughly one in four Americans do absolutely no physical activity at all. This is concerning because it means that many of us are unable to do the basic activities that our daily lives require. For example, a 2007 survey done by the LA Fitness gym chain showed that half of those surveyed couldn't even touch their toes. Further, 68 percent of the surveyed population were unable to do twenty sit-ups, 58 percent couldn't cycle for twenty minutes and 42 percent couldn't climb three flights of stairs without getting out of breath. My hunch is that if this survey were to be repeated at the time this book was written (2024), the results would be even worse. If this sounds like an isolated problem that only affects the unfit, it definitely isn't.

Outside of the personal risks to physical health and longevity, the consequences of physical inactivity on a larger scale are dire. The Citadel conducted a survey in 2019 with the US Army's Defense Centers for Public Health–Aberdeen and the AHA. What they found was that 27 percent of potential enlistees aged seventeen to twenty-four were too obese or overweight, to qualify for military service. Obesity aside, the study also revealed that 47 percent of men and 59 percent of women failed the Army's entry-level fitness training test. Sure enough, the percentage of eligible recruits who exceed the percent-body-fat standards for the US Military as a whole has doubled for men and tripled for women since 1960. Experts warn that our military readiness is severely compromised as a result. Certainly, these inadequacies in our population carry over to other important roles in our society as well. There are similar fitness test requirements for law enforcement officers, firefighters, paramedics, search and rescue professionals, etc.

And what about jobs that carry a high physical burden by requiring heavy lifting and physical endurance, such as construction work? What will happen when we don't have enough people who are fit enough for these roles? It turns out that being "athletically pathetic" as a collective population can have some pretty grave consequences.

Chapter 2

The Benefits of Exercise and Physical Activity

It is health that is real wealth and not pieces of gold and silver.
—Mahatma Gandhi

Everyone knows that exercise is good for you. But just how good is it? Exercise has many benefits. Beyond minimizing your risk of dying early or developing diseases, of which some of the most serious being heart disease, stroke, diabetes, and certain types of cancer, exercise can benefit your health in ways you might have never imagined. Not only can exercise help you manage your weight, strengthen your bones and muscles, and improve your brain health, it can also improve your sleep, sex, skin health, reproductive health, and overall physical resilience. Being in good physical shape can even boost your chances of survival and recovery from accidents, injuries, and illness. For many people with a chronic disease, exercise can help manage, ameliorate and even cure their disease. This can be especially true for mental illnesses, metabolic diseases, and conditions that cause chronic pain. Regular physical activity can also help people with disabilities by contributing to the maintenance—and even improvement—of their ability to carry out daily living activities and supporting their independence to the maximum extent possible.

Our brains love exercise

Exercise can preserve and improve your brain health in many ways. As we age, our brains have a tendency to slow down or experience cognitive decline. This impairment of the brain can be caused by a variety of factors responsible for dementia such as is seen in Alzheimer's, Parkinson's, and Huntington's diseases. Studies in both mice and humans have shown that long-term exercise can delay the onset of this cognitive decline and help with the symptoms of people who have already been diagnosed.

Physical activity stimulates brain chemicals that promote happiness and relaxation, helping to hedge against feelings of stress, depression, and anxiety that are common in our society. The effects of exercise can also lead to an overall boost in mood and an improvement in confidence, self-esteem, and overall energy levels. A short bout of exercise has been noted as one of the most effective techniques to enhance mood in healthy people. Study subjects showed decreases in tension, depression, anger, and confusion. Long-term exercise habits have shown even more interesting results in studies using mice. These results showed that habitual or long-term exercise produces effects against anxiety and depression at similar or greater levels than medications used to treat these problems!

A 2017 review by Julia Basso and Wendy Suzuki in the journal *Brain Plasticity* noted that the effects of exercise can increase attention, long-term memory, recollection, reward-based learning, and motor functions. These benefits might help enhance performance in work or school-related tasks.

The continuation of clinical studies will be important in determining how beneficial regular physical activity can be in preventing the cognitive decline that occurs with age as well as treating other psychological and behavioral conditions such as attention-deficit hyperactivity disorder (ADHD), schizophrenia, and post-traumatic stress disorders.

Exercise and the bedroom

Exercise can help you fall asleep more quickly and get a longer, more restful sleep. In response to exercise, the brain releases melatonin, a hormone that regulates sleep-wake cycles. Since stress is a common barrier to falling and staying asleep, exercise helps sleep by reducing stress and increasing feelings of relaxation. What's more, the increases in energy expenditure and body temperature during exercise help the body's restorative processes and lower body temperature during sleep, which in turn, improves sleep quality.

Both aerobic and resistance training improve sleep quality. Further, these benefits extend to those with sleep disorders. In a 2012 systematic review lead by Yang Pei-Yu in *The Journal of Physiology*, adults aged forty and older with sleep problems were studied over ten to fourteen weeks while they regularly engaged in a formal exercise training program consisting of either aerobic or resistance exercise. In addition to an improvement in sleep quality, the results showed a decrease in difficulty and time falling asleep and a decrease in the need for sleep aid medications.

But sleep isn't the only bedroom activity that can improve with exercise. Regular physical activity can also enhance your sex life. Since exercise has been shown to strengthen the heart, promote circulation, and improve the tone and flexibility of skeletal muscles, these benefits translate into better sex. Sexual desire, performance, pleasure, and frequency have all been proven in scientific studies to be positively impacted by regular exercise. Exercise also improves sexual function in post-menopausal women, women with polycystic ovary disease, and even men with erectile dysfunction. In a study by Isis Begot in the *American Journal of Cardiology*, forty-one male cardiac patients were prescribed a progressive walking program that could be done from their homes four times per week for thirty days. After the thirty days, the men reported a 71 percent improvement in their erectile dysfunction symptoms.

Add exercise to your skin care regimen

If that isn't exciting enough, did you know that exercise can improve the appearance of aging skin? Regular moderate exercise increases your body's production of natural antioxidants. Antioxidants help protect the body's cells, keeping them functioning like they did when you were younger. In addition, exercise helps promote good blood flow, including to the skin and muscles, and induces skin cell adaptations that slow the aging process of skin cells.

Drive to survive

What about exercising regularly enough and long enough to achieve fitness? What, exactly, is fitness and why do you need it? The *Oxford English Dictionary* defines fitness in biology as an organism's ability to survive and reproduce in a particular environment. Let that term *survive* ring louder. In nature, most animals need to be fit in order to survive! They have to be able to hunt and forage for their food and water, find and build shelter to keep them safe, and escape from predators and danger. In nature, animals use fitness to select their mates to reproduce the next generation of their species. As humans have evolved, the connection between fitness and survivability has faded slightly. But it still has a great deal of relevance.

Contrary to the requirements of our not-so-distance ancestors, most of us no longer have the need or motivation to grow, farm, forage, or hunt for our own food in order to survive—activities which require a great deal of physical fitness. But we do need, at a bare minimum, the ability to lift a Costco-sized flat of canned food in and out of a shopping cart, the strength to drag a heavy trash can across a driveway, or put an overstuffed suitcase in the overhead bin of an airplane (provided a stranger doesn't offer to do it for you). Practical applications for fitness are everywhere in our daily lives, and life's basic tasks are a lot easier when you're fit.

While not always top-of-mind for everyone, nor in every season of life, reproduction is still vital to the survival of the human species. Our human brains subconsciously choose mates based on their fitness to reproduce and to raise children. Despite our social efforts to paint beauty on fashion models who are too thin or too heavy, the fact remains that fertility in both males and females is optimal in people who carry a healthy weight and project an image of fitness to bear and raise children. Our subconscious minds attract us to healthy-looking people for a reason. And certainly a parent's ability to chase after a toddler is strictly dependent on their ability to run! The constant demands of picking up, holding, and carrying small children present a physical challenge even for seasoned athletes. The ability to adequately care for and raise children is, especially in the early years, very dependent on physical abilities. Further, the health and fitness examples that we set for children as they grow will determine their standard for health later in their lives. Our abilities to have and raise healthy children is largely dependent on our fitness to do so.

Have you ever imagined yourself in a crisis? A fire, natural disaster, or a physical attack? Would you be fit enough to survive and escape? Could you quickly climb out the window of a burning car after a crash . . . with a broken leg? Could you run down several flights of stairs with a child in your arms? What if someone were chasing you? These all sound like things only first responders should train for. But what happens before 911 is called? The truth in many cases is that you're on your own. Your baseline fitness levels in situations such as these can mean the difference between life and death. Being in good physical shape saves your life in accidents. A strong framework of bones, muscles, and circulatory system are great attributions to physical durability in crisis situations.

A nudge toward physical resilience

If survival of an accident or injury weren't enough, being physically fit can also help you effectively recover and heal. People who are considered physically fit heal more rapidly from infections, injury, and surgery than inactive people. One possible reason for this is that fit people are less likely to experience pain because of a reduced sensitivity of pain receptors in the brain and a reduction in inflammatory components in the blood. This increased healing ability was well demonstrated during the COVID-19 pandemic. People who were physically inactive prior to infection were much more likely to be hospitalized and/or to die from COVID-19 than active people were. I can personally attest to the increased capacity to heal as it relates to fitness levels after successfully healing from the birth to two children and four abdominal surgeries within a seven-year window. The more physically fit I was at the time of these events, the quicker I recovered. Physical fitness has indeed helped me survive and thrive though many of my own life challenges.

Feel-good benefits

Of course, all of the benefits already discussed here are backed by science and could be considered textbook examples. But if you ask people who have a regular exercise routine about the positive impacts they've experienced, you'll get a whole different warm and fuzzy perspective. They'll tell you things like

- "I've formed lifelong friendships at my gym."
- "The community in my fitness classes keeps me motivated."
- "I thought I had reached the edge of my physical capabilities, but then I was able to do so much more that I surprised myself."
- "My fitness routine has taught me a lot about myself and has made me a better person."
- "I accomplished things that I never thought my body was capable of doing."
- "My fitness routine has helped me heal traumas of my past and given me a new sense of pride and confidence."
- "I finally feel great, and I look good naked!"

If exercise sounds like a magic bullet and the answer to many of life's problems, that's because it is. If you aren't keen on requiring a metric ton of actual medicine for the rest of your life, then you should get comfortable with the idea that exercise *is* medicine. There is still a lot of research to be done in order to understand all of the health benefits of exercise and physical fitness. But with what we know now, it is entirely possible that exercise is more effective than pills and other medical interventions at keeping us living longer, healthier lives. But how much movement do we need exactly? And which type? The next chapter addresses these questions in detail.

Chapter 3
What Is Exercise and Physical Activity?

An inch of movement will bring you closer to your goals than a mile of intention.
—Steve Maraboli

There are four factors to consider when thinking about the movement you need on a regular basis to be fit and healthy:

1. The intensity of activity
2. The type of the activity
3. The frequency of the activity
4. The duration of the activity

Not all exercise is created equal, so these details are important to note.

The intensity of the activity

What actually counts as exercise or physical activity? Most activity is classified as having light, moderate, or vigorous intensities. These intensity classifications are based on the average adult using a sedentary starting point. Exercise scientists gauge the intensity of an activity by the amount of effort or energy the activity takes to perform. This energy is measured by what is called a metabolic equivalent or MET. One MET is equal to the amount of oxygen a person requires while sitting quietly at rest. The measurement of a MET takes into account a person's weight during a one-minute snapshot of their activity. Another way to gauge the intensity of an activity is to use heart rate. While this method can seem a bit more complicated for some, it is just another way to explain an increase in oxygen requirements. Because our bodies need more oxygen to carry out an activity, our heart rate must increase to deliver it more quickly to the working parts of our body. To keep things simple, we are only going to discuss the intensity of physical activity in terms of our bodies' need for oxygen—our METs. It is important to note that since METs account for a person's weight, someone carrying excess weight will likely have increased oxygen requirements. This means they will likely experience a higher intensity and fatigue of exercise more quickly and prominently than a person who is not carrying excess weight.

Have you ever started climbing a flight of stairs and noticed how your lungs are huffing and puffing to help you to the top? This is your body's need for more oxygen during your climb. For most people, walking up stairs is considered a moderate-intensity activity. This is because your body needs more oxygen to climb stairs than it needs to get up to slowly walk across a room, which is (or should be) a light-intensity activity.

Light-intensity activities are activities that require less than three METs. Because your body requires less oxygen during light-intensity activities, these are activities that you can usually carry out while breathing through your nose with your mouth closed or even while singing a song. Examples of light-intensity activities include slow and comfortable walking, preparing food, making a bed, and washing dishes. Light-intensity activity is what I like to call "non-exercise exercise." It is performing simple daily living tasks that require movement without intentional exertion.

Now you may be thinking that if light-intensity activity isn't formal exercise, then it doesn't count for anything, right?

Wrong!

When it comes to losing weight and maintaining a healthy lifestyle, light-intensity activity can make a huge difference. In fact, when it comes to losing weight, these activities can often account for the majority of the results because they are the types of activities that can be done for the longest duration with the least amount of effort. Experts call this type of activity NEAT (non-exercise activity thermogenesis). This is basically a fancy term to explain the metabolic benefits gained and the calories burned by the casual activities you do in your life outside of sleeping, eating, and intentional exercise.

Moderate-intensity activities use more METs than light-intensity activities. These activities require between three and six METs. Because moderate-intensity activity increases your body's need for oxygen, you will usually be forced to breathe through your mouth instead of your nose and lose the ability to sing during these activities. However, you will know you are doing something of moderate intensity but not vigorous intensity if you can still carry on a conversation with a friend. Examples of moderate-intensity activities are brisk walking, washing windows, slow dancing, and vacuuming.

Vigorous-intensity activities are those that require six or more METs and the highest amount of oxygen to carry out. You will know you are engaged in a vigorous-intensity activity if you are breathing heavily through your mouth and cannot carry on a conversation. I personally know when I've reached this level of intensity when I can say nothing more than a couple of four-letter words with exasperation.

Most intentional exercise can be switched between moderate and vigorous intensities. For example, lifting light weights slowly can be a moderate-intensity activity while, in contrast, lifting heavy weights quickly can be more vigorous. Your fitness levels will ultimately determine what intensity an activity is for you. A slow two-minute jog for me is a moderate-intensity activity because I am an avid runner. For my overweight, out-of-shape, sedentary neighbor, a two-minute jog at the same pace could be vigorous.

Movement is very much a use-it-or-lose-it skill. This is why I haven't been able to do the splits since I was a ten-year-old gymnast. If you aren't constantly teaching your body that it must do a certain activity, your body will not easily do that activity when the time becomes necessary. While stretching exercises are valuable, the splits aren't necessary or important to me, so I stopped doing them. When I tried a hot yoga class for the first time at the age of thirty-eight, I swore my legs were going to snap clean off at the hips. Nothing truly compares to the sensation of experiencing sharp groin pain while sweating into your eyeballs and breathing in pungent foot odor in 103 degree temperatures. So as you might guess, hot yoga is not my activity of choice. Certainly, we all can't be in top physical shape to do everything—that isn't the goal. The goal is to be in the best physical shape possible to live a long and healthy life doing the things that are necessary and important to us.

The type of the activity

Naturally, the type of physical activity matters in relation to the intensity. While yoga is an excellent exercise for flexibility and balance, it is not usually the best choice if you want to increase cardiovascular endurance or calorie expenditure for weight loss; a better choice to achieve these goals would be a regular and intentional moderate- to vigorous-intensity activity coupled with an increase in NEAT.

Intentional exercise is usually separated into three distinct buckets: aerobic (cardio), strength training, and balance and flexibility. Aerobic exercises are activities that get you breathing hard enough to bring you into the moderate- or vigorous-intensity categories. These are activities such as walking at a fast pace, swimming, running, cycling, dancing, and tennis. Strength training exercises are activities that build strength for certain muscles or groups of muscles. Examples of these types of exercises are lifting weights, body weight exercises (such as push-ups, pull-ups, or sit-ups), Pilates, or resistance band exercises. Strength training can also be done in a way that brings you into the moderate- or vigorous-intensity categories as well, adding some cardiovascular benefits. Balance and flexibility exercises include movements done during yoga, tai chi, and stretching. These are usually lighter in intensity but can often be ramped up to a moderate intensity and sometimes vigorous intensity.

Many exercise activities and sports can span the entire intensity spectrum and provide benefits in more than one way. For example, synchronized swimming—or water ballet—is exercise that increases balance and flexibility as well as cardiovascular endurance and muscle strength. One routine can span the entire intensity spectrum. The point here is that different types of physical activity can have different classifications and therefore yield different results. The type, duration, and intensity of which exercise you do will matter in relation to your goals. I discuss fitness goals and the details of how to reach them in Chapter 7.

The duration and frequency of the activity

The CDC and the US Department of Health and Human Services say that adults need 150 minutes of moderate-intensity physical activity or 75 minutes of vigorous aerobic activity and two days of muscle strengthening activity per week. If you prefer moderate cardio, this can be broken down into three fifty-minute sessions per week or five thirty-minute cardio sessions per week. If vigorous cardio is more your style, you can break it down into five fifteen-minute cardio sessions per week or three twenty-five-minute cardio sessions. This is just a generic prescription for what an average person needs on a weekly basis. To me, this represents a baseline and a bare minimum requirement for health. It does not take into consideration what a person would need in order to gain twenty pounds of muscle or lose thirty pounds of fat. And you might have noticed that it completely neglects to include exercises to improve balance and flexibility, which are crucial aspects of fitness. Like all prescriptions, the intensity, type, frequency, and duration of exercise should be tailored to the individual and their goals. In medicine, we tailor prescriptions for age, weight, gender, disease, and many other factors. No two people on this planet are the same, so therefore it would seem ludicrous to assume that everyone needs the exact same prescription for physical activity. As a general rule, the more you move your body, the better the result, barring that you aren't putting yourself at risk of injury.

All of the topics covered in these first three chapters serve as helpful information to keep in your back pocket. Maybe you learned something helpful or maybe you already knew it all. But more than likely, learning or knowing all this information isn't going to be enough to motivate you to into a new and different active lifestyle. *Knowing* that something is good for you isn't always enough to make you *do* that thing. Heck, even *wanting* to do the things that are good for you isn't always enough. In Chapter 4, we talk about why.

Chapter 4

Why Is the Exercise Habit So Hard?

Tough times never last, but tough people do.
—Robert H. Schuller

Exercise is hard. Regular exercise is even harder. If it weren't, you wouldn't have bought a book to convince yourself to do it. There are a lot things we should be doing (and not doing) for our health that are too difficult for us to get on board with. We're told to get enough sleep, but we stay up late anyway to finish our Netflix binge. We're told to eat less junk food, but those potato chips and desserts are just so tasty.

We aren't naturally inclined to exercise

During my last year in pharmacy school, I worked with a man who underwent a surgical above-the-knee amputation on one of his legs due to poorly controlled diabetes. He flat out told me that he was prepared to lose his other leg to the effects of his disease because he was unwilling to monitor his blood sugar levels and take insulin. His stubbornness and apathy were astounding to me at the time, but I soon learned they aren't uncommonly seen in the medical field. Making healthy lifestyle changes is actually really hard for people to do on a permanent basis. But *why* is it so hard? Why do we defy our health recommendations when we know better?

On the most primal level, intentional exercise is not a natural inclination for human beings. That is to say, we didn't evolve to get up early in the morning and go to spin class five days a week. Early human beings got their exercise passively through labor activities. They gathered materials, built shelter, and foraged and hunted for food. Because life presented many periods of food scarcity, the body's natural tendency was driven toward conserving its energy. This meant that spending energy on physical activity would have had to have been worth the reward. For our early ancestors, if physical activity didn't earn them survival tokens in the form of food, water, shelter, or safety, they were better served by sitting by the fire and chatting with their pals.

More recently (but still twelve thousand years ago), humans began transitioning to agricultural means of obtaining food, which made their work more energy efficient. Sure, herding sheep and planting crops were labor intensive, but the rewards generally made it worth the effort in terms of energy expenditure. Finally, we arrived at the industrial age, during which machines replaced muscle, and we traded farms for factories.

These technological advances and changes in the ways we survived happened far more quickly than the human species' ability to evolve and adapt. It is simply no longer pertinent in this day and age for large swaths of the population to perform physically laborious tasks in order to survive, but our bodies don't know it. While our environments in the developed world are a stark difference to how things looked twelve thousand years ago, our bodies still largely exist structurally and physiologically as they did in the age of the hunter-gatherers —and they are still wired to conserve energy (and also consume it!) as if food sources were frequently scarce. In many parts of the world where food is in fact scarce, this wiring is still quite relevant and necessary for survival. In Western society, however, it is working against us in a big way.

Not only is the human body naturally inclined to conserve energy but also to do what is easy and to take the path of least resistance. More bluntly, we are hard-wired for laziness. Why else would we so quickly and enthusiastically develop and adopt all of the technology that makes our lives exponentially easier? A study published in eLife conducted by researchers at the University College London and the National Institute of Information and Communications Technology in Japan found that humans naturally and subconsciously pick the path of least resistance even if the easier decision is not the best or the correct one. This highlights the idea that any activity we perceive as challenging is automatically less appealing to us even if we know the activity is necessary and important. This also shows that human beings are hardwired to conserve cognitive (or brain) energy just as readily as physical energy.

. . .

We chase instant gratification

Our bodies are designed to conserve mental and physical energy, but we are also hardwired to prioritize things that provide instant gratification. Human nature dictates that when we perform activities that reward us with immediate pleasure, we will be more highly motivated to perform those activities. Sigmund Freud popularized this concept more than 120 years ago with a theory called the pleasure principle. The pleasure principle explains how human behavior is dictated by the instincts that satisfy basic human needs. For example, thirst is your body's natural cue to drink water, which is a basic need for survival. When you are thirsty and you drink water, you feel immediate pleasure and satisfaction. This pattern repeats for other basic survival needs such as food, sleep, and sex.

Dopamine is the chemical in our brain that is released to make us feel that powerful rush of pleasure after we satisfy our needs. This is why dopamine is also the brain chemical responsible for addictions to things such as food, sex, and social media. It gives us a feeling of satisfaction that can be greatly intensified for certain things in certain people. Some people feel this type of intense satisfaction after exercise (sometimes called "runner's high"), which might explain why exercise can be so helpful for those living with depression and why exercise addiction exists at all. However, many of us don't feel a sense of instant gratification after one workout—especially because one workout will not produce instant weight loss and six-pack abs.

It is because exercise lacks this ability to produce instant gratification that is so difficult to habitually perform. You brush your teeth and your mouth feels instantly clean.

You get a lot of likes on social media and you feel instantly liked and accepted in your social circle. But if you go outside and run two miles, you might just feel instantly sweaty, winded, and tired. Further, for most people, exercise does not carry (consciously or subconsciously) the same prioritization as other basic needs such as water, food, and sleep. Therefore, your body is not routinely prompting you to habitually exercise the way it is with sensations of thirst, hunger, or exhaustion. Exercise not only lacks the built-in reward of instant gratification but the cue to initiate the activity in the first place, inevitably pushing it lower on your priority list. After all, if a specific action isn't going to reward you with instant pleasure—and you don't need it to survive in the short term—it is easy to pass off as unnecessary.

There is pain in the gain

The opposite side of the pleasure principle coin is the natural instinct to avoid activities that cause pain and discomfort. Pain is the body's natural cue to avoid activities that may cause injury. For most people, exercise (especially if you are out of practice) can be extremely uncomfortable and even painful. So the natural inclination is to avoid it altogether. What is worse, the longer your body exists in a sedentary state without exposure to exercise, the more painful and difficult it becomes to initiate or reinitiate exercise activities, especially when you don't ease into it slowly. This happens even to the fittest people and can be such a strong deterrent that it can easily derail an exercise routine that was in place for a while before, say, an illness or a vacation occurred.

To summarize, habitual, intentional exercise is difficult for modern human beings because we aren't biologically wired to seek it out. Our brains and bodies evolved to conserve energy and only engage in activities that passively contribute to our survival in a manner we deem worthwhile. Our subconscious mind automatically assigns and prioritizes activities that require the least amount of physical and mental energy, avoid any pain or discomfort, and offer instant rewards. So if you want to make a legitimate, science-based excuse for why you don't have a good exercise routine, you can just chalk it up to good ol' human nature.

Chapter 5
Common Reasons for Failing to Permanently Adopt an Exercise Routine

The greatest glory in living lies not in never failing, but in rising every time we fail.
—Nelson Mandela

You can certainly blame your failure to achieve fitness success on human nature. But what else can you blame? Understanding your failures on a deeper level can be empowering because it gives you the opportunity to focus on how and why you failed. Pinning down the problem makes it easier to figure out how to fix it and then try again with a fresh perspective. This chapter is going to address common reasons for failing to permanently adopt the exercise habit.

Mama said . . .

Extensive clinical research and countless studies have

Caitlyn Tanner, Pharm.D

found strong links between our parents' (or primary caregivers') behaviors during our childhood and how we act as adults. The examples our parents set for us can be responsible for forming our adult habits and behaviors in nearly every area of our lives. The importance of our parents' conscious and subconscious influences that we carry into adulthood cannot be overstated. The behavioral examples of our parents impose a profound impact on our adult identities, effecting a wide variety of behaviors from how we interact in relationships, to how we manage our finances, to our diet and exercise habits. Studies have even linked parental influence in childhood to mental and physical health all the way through adulthood. If exercise and physical health were not positively modeled for you during your childhood, you most certainly are not alone. New studies continue to investigate just how strong your parents' influence actually is on your diet and exercise habits. In fact, a recent 2022 study published by JMIR Formative Research showed that parental encouragement of children to consume fruits and vegetables in their diets and perform physical activity had a very strong impact on their children. Most interestingly was that the maternal influence was shown to be the strongest and most limiting factor in promoting a healthy lifestyle for the children in the study.

As a pharmacist, many of my patients have attempted to convince me that obesity and all of its associated negative health effects simply runs in their family and that genetics are 100 percent to blame. While there are certainly strong genetic components to our own human anatomy, physiology, and predispositions to disease, to ignore lifestyle and poor habits entirely is neglecting to see the forest for the tress. Diet and activity levels usually constitute the bulk of the issue. An entire family of five obese people is nearly always an entire family who shares the same poor diet and sedentary lifestyle habits.

To look at your childhood and familial or social influences with a critical eye in an attempt to identify a problem can indeed be daunting and often painful. The goal is not to place blame but rather to reach realization about why certain habits, such as that of regular exercise, were not ingrained into your value system and might still be imposing a negative influence on you today. I was lucky to be raised by a mother who modeled regular exercise. As a child, I spent many hours in a children's play area while my mom took Jazzercise classes. And I remember that her running shoes never stayed new for long. She often forced my brother and me outside on nice days to run in the yard, to play tag with the neighborhood kids, or to ride our bikes to the park. Certainly this had a lasting impact on me on both a conscious and subconscious level, priming me for an active adult lifestyle.

If you weren't raised to incorporate regular physical activity into your life, starting and sticking with an exercise routine could be all the more difficult because it was not ingrained in your value system during the most crucial phases of your brain development. But with focus and dedication, this can be overcome. It is never too late to adopt new, positive values and habits and pass them on to future generations. If you don't come from a fit family, a fit family can come from you.

. . .

Blending in with your surroundings

While we're on the topic of values and setting good examples, an obligatory mention of your social group remains in order. What do your friends and acquaintances do for fun? Are they fit? Do they routinely coax you into unhealthy habits like eating out frequently, doing sedentary activities, or having a few too many adult beverages? Maybe all of the above. You may have heard this quote made popular by motivational speaker Jim Rohn: "You are the average of the five people you spend the most time with." The truth to this statement has been heavily debated online. However, the influence of the people in your life should be given adequate consideration when it comes to your health. It is possible that the influence of your social circle has created some road blocks to getting fit in the past. I talk more about the importance of social influence in Chapter 7.

Doing the wrong thing in the wrong place with the wrong people

Arguably the most obvious reason why you might have previously failed to stick to a fitness routine is that you're simply doing it all wrong (or at least wrong for you)! This may come as a surprise, but exercise isn't really supposed to be complete physical or mental torture. If it has consistently felt like torture, that's a clue that you're definitely doing it wrong.

How do I know this? Because I did it wrong too.

After graduating high school and being catapulted into adulthood, I lost almost all of the structure that I once had in my daily activities. A regular daily schedule and the organized pressure of participating in school and club sports all came to a screeching halt. Like a light switch, the minute I started college, I immediately became sedentary and gained at least the freshman fifteen.

So what did I do about it? I joined a gym, of course. A regular, big-box "Globo Gym" (*Dodgeball*, anyone?) complete with a thousand machines (most of which I had no idea how to use), floor-to-ceiling mirrors, a scan card, and a free month of membership with an annual contract. I showed up for my first workout by myself, stared across the open floor of exercise equipment and people who looked like they knew what they were doing, and then made a beeline straight for a treadmill—the only machine that I *thought* I might know how to use.

After pushing a bunch of buttons, I finally got the thing going and started walking. This was the only thing I knew how to do while I thought about what the heck else I was supposed to be doing in this place to stop getting so fat. I walked for a very long time while studying what other people were doing for their exercise. Some of these people looked very fit and very confident about what they were doing, which lit a little fire of anxiety in my chest. Over the next several months and what eventually turned into years, I learned what most of the machinery was for and how to ignore what everyone else was doing while staying out of people's way. Even with music in my headphones, I was desperately bored and annoyed with what I was doing because it was being done fairly randomly, with no specific purpose, plan, guidance, or direction—and I hated every minute of it. For several consecutive Januarys, I experienced the New Year's gym rush and had to wait for thirty or more minutes for a weight or cardio machine. And the worst part was, I neither lost the weight nor got in shape doing what I was doing at that Globo Gym.

So I eventually gave up on it. I don't mean to say that big-box gyms are bad in any way. Their mere existence is upheld by the demand people have for convenient, reasonably-priced, self-directed ways to exercise. But if you've ever had an experience like mine, in which you tried to find a simple and obvious solution to your lack of fitness but failed miserably, it might be because you're doing it wrong too.

It took a lot of extra tries, creativity, self-reflection, and even more frustration after the Globo Gym failure before I figured out why I was unable to successfully jump onto a fitness routine. To boil down what happened, I was doing the wrong activities at the wrong places with the wrong people and, most importantly, with the wrong mindset. In my desperate attempt to get in shape and stop growing around the midsection, I hadn't even considered that there were at least fifteen different ways to skin this cat that could have provided for a better outcome. And I wallowed in that failure for far too long. Chapters 6 through 9 explain in more detail how to best set yourself up for success so you don't have to quit your Globo Gym for the fifteenth time.

Trapped in a cycle

This is going to seem off topic so just stay with me for a

minute. Did you know that ants sometimes walk in a continuous rotating circle? A phenomenon called an ant mill happens when a group of army ants are separated from their main foraging group. The ants lose their scent track and begin to follow one another, forming a continuous rotating circle. This circle is known as a "death spiral" because the ants will often walk in this circle until they eventually die of exhaustion. In a similar framework, another reason people fail to adopt a regular exercise routine is what I have coined "death trap cycles." These are cycles of feelings and behaviors that take you around and around through negative stop points until you die, making it extremely difficult to change your trajectory. The main cause of being stuck in a death trap cycle is poor mental health and mindset.

Let's take depression as an example. A quickly growing epidemic across the world, depression simplified is a mental health disorder that causes a loss of pleasure or interest in usually enjoyable activities and can be marked by strong feelings of sadness, hopelessness, and pessimism. A person who is in the throes of depression might feel it's impossible to get out of bed and go for a brisk walk due to a lack of mental and physical energy. But we know from our discussion in Chapter 2 that exercise can be a powerful tool in fighting depression, and it actually helps improve energy levels. So a depressed person may stay sedentary, possibly becoming or remaining obese. And obesity and sedentary lifestyles are known factors that contribute to depression, so therein lies the cycle.

No matter where a person started in the cycle, forcing the body into intentional physical movement is one of the best ways out. Other death trap cycles that can co-exist with depression and other mental health disorders are the cycles of poor self-esteem and poor self-confidence. People with low self-esteem or self-confidence genuinely feel they are too out of shape or too overweight, leading to feelings of intimidation toward going to a gym or fitness facility. So they don't go and predictably become more overweight and out of shape only to arrive back at the same excuse for not engaging in regular exercise. Again, the best way out of this cycle is to force your way out and into an exercise habit, which brings me to the topic of excuses . . .

Excuses, excuses

You knew it was coming, I'm sure. It's high time to place some blame on your excuses. The ultimate excuse for failing to get fit in the past is your own excuses! We all make them for one reason or another. The point of an excuse is to excuse poor behavior and/or to excuse yourself from a responsibility you have to yourself and others. Making excuses is a behavior far worse than whining because it provides justification for your failures, not just a simple expression of dissatisfaction. Excuses actually set you free, or at least you may *feel* liberated by making them. When it comes to exercise, I estimate that well over 95 percent of all excuses are hollow and provide no valid reason to free yourself entirely from doing what you should to get in shape. Chapter 4 discussed why exercise is so hard, so naturally we are all going to have lots of excuses to avoid it. But excuses never serve us well, and overcoming our excuses is paramount to our own success.

I'm certainly no stranger to excuses myself. I'm only human. In fact, I've been a victim to my own excuses more times than I'd like to admit. Looking back, nearly every excuse I accepted in my fitness life was a snapshot of a time I gave up on myself. To prove it to you, I've compiled a list of all my pathetic excuses for avoiding exercise to share with you in this book. I hope you're ready because here they are:

- I'm too tired.
- I don't have enough time.
- My shoulder hurts.
- My foot hurts.
- My knee hurts.
- My butt hurts.
- My [insert any one of 8000 body parts] hurts.
- I have a hangnail.
- I'm wearing a Band-Aid.
- It's too cold.
- It's too windy.
- It's too hot.
- I should rest.
- I have to do laundry.
- My kids need me to stay home.
- I had a long day at work.
- I had a hard week.
- My favorite show is on TV.
- It's going to rain.
- My car is broken.
- My clothes don't fit.

- I'm fat and my thighs rub together.
- The gym is too expensive.
- I have more important things to do.
- It's too far.
- I'm going to be late.
- The traffic is bad.
- I feel sad.
- I have a pimple.
- I have a headache.
- My shoes are worn down.
- My body isn't designed for this.
- I'll never get in shape anyway.
- I'm still recovering from that bad cold I had in 1998.
- I have lady problems.
- I have gas.
- I JUST. CAN'T.
- I was invited to this other thing that seems a lot more fun.
- I'd rather be doing anything but exercise.
- I'm hungry.
- I ate too much.
- I can't find my water bottle or my gym bag.
- I'm too ugly for public display.
- I just took a shower.
- There is a war in Ukraine.
- My dog ate my underwear. (Yes, this actually happened. He survived.)

Well, that was embarrassing. And to admit that I hung my hat on many of those to skip workouts and throw away my goals feels shameful. Every last one of those excuses delayed my fitness success, sabotaged my health, and kept me believing that my comfort was more important than my personal growth. In fact, the worst and longest-running excuse I ever made started in my twenties. I enjoyed running and had even completed a half-marathon when I was twenty-two. Several of my friends had put a bug in my ear that I should run a marathon. To me, 26.2 miles (42 kilometers) seemed a ridiculous distance and completely unattainable. I was consumed with self-doubt and intimidation. For over fifteen years I told everyone, including myself, that the joints in my feet were bad, I was recommended for bunion surgery, and that there was no way my bone and joint structure would sustain such grueling training over such long distances. It was partly true. I do have bad feet.

But after bouncing back from a couple of surprise abdominal surgeries in my mid-thirties, I decided to finally tell myself the truth—I could never be certain that I was truly incapable of something that I had never even tried. So I actually did try, and I succeeded in running not one, but two complete 26.2-mile marathons in the years leading up to my fortieth birthday with healthy feet through all. Excuses are the tools we use to give up on our dreams and goals. They distract us from our full potential and make us believe that we can't make—or we aren't worth—the effort. Excuses wipe out good intentions and ideas that have the potential to change our lives for the better.

Hopefully you can identify with some of what was discussed in this chapter on a personal level. Diagnosing the reasons for past failures allows us to pave the road to future success. If you can now identify that (1) you have people in your life (past and present) who might not have positively influenced you, (2) you've been doing it all wrong, (3) you've spent some time in a death trap cycle, and/or (4) you're making too many excuses, then congratulations! As Steve Jobs said, "If you define the problem correctly, you almost have the solution". The next chapters will help you ease into the solution.

Chapter 6
Mind Over Matter

You don't have to control your thoughts. You just have to stop letting them control you.
—Dan Millman

Sports psychologists often tout success in athletics as 90 percent mental and only 10 percent physical. The numbers are easily debatable, but most can agree that fitness is much more than 50 percent psychological. Were it less, there would likely be no such thing as a sports psychologist. The way we allow our thought processes to affect exercise and fitness training matters a great deal. On the surface, we avoid activities that are uncomfortable, which can cause negative thoughts to pervade said activities. But there are ways around this reaction. If we can re-think some of our default thought processes surrounding exercise, we can become just as mentally fit as we can physically. Mental and physical strength and endurance go hand in hand. Once mental fitness is truly realized, physical fitness follows much more easily. Reframing our thought processes about fitness and exercise is one of the most pertinent aspects of fitness success.

Be stronger than your excuses

We can start by revisiting the topic of excuses. I place excuses into two categories: Category One excuses and Category Two excuses.

A Category One excuse is an excuse with a heavy amount of cow manure and is sometimes an outright lie you are using for self-sabotage. A Category Two excuse is an excuse with an opportunity to find a solution, so you can pivot. Taking my own list of excuses as an example, excuses such as "my body isn't designed for this" is a category One excuse. I told myself that lie for fifteen years only to find that by body is not only designed for running but it can actually excel at it.

When Category One excuses are bald-faced lies, you can easily ask a couple questions to catch yourself. "I'll never get in shape anyway" is a good example. Ask yourself questions like

- How do I know this is true and accurate?
- Am I lying to myself because I don't want to work out?
- Would I say this to my best friend about his/her workout?

With a couple quick minutes of self-reflection, you will usually know you are giving up on yourself with this kind of excuse. Category One excuses can also be easily squashed with a simple phrase: Suck it up, Buttercup! Excuses like, "I'd rather be doing anything other than exercise" and "I had a long day at work" are Category One excuses perfect for sucking it up and getting on with it.

Category Two excuses are those that might be true and legitimate but have easy solutions—sometimes multiple solutions. Here are a few examples:

Excuse: I just took a shower.

Solution: Smell good at the gym and then take another one.

Excuse: My shoes are worn down and my feet hurt.

Solution: Suck it up one last time and then buy new shoes as a reward. (Or go for a swim instead.) (Or do calisthenics in bare feet at home as a substitute.)

Excuse: The weather is bad.

Solution: Swap something in your calendar and reschedule! (Or do an online calisthenics workout at home.) (Or suck it up and run in the rain like a champ.)

Excuse: I have gas.

Solution: Take a straw and a Gas-X and suck it up! (And exercise might help anyway.)

As you can see, Category One and Category Two excuses can share some overlap. But the bottom line is that you can make progress, or you can make excuses, but you can't make both. You *have* to call yourself out. Is your excuse really worth more to you than your success?

Now you might be saying, "but wait, I have a *real* excuse!"

These are Category Three excuses.

What are Category Three excuses? Probably less than 5 percent of all excuses. Maybe you are recovering from childbirth, surgery, a bad accident, or a death in your family. Those are indeed real excuses that can put a stop to any fitness routine. It's OK to take a break when you need to as long as you don't make any Category One or Category Two excuses to extend your time off longer than necessary (like that bad cold from 1998 that I'm still recovering from). Remember that exercise is *good* for you! It can heal you physically, mentally, and emotionally. If you lose the will to get back in the game after a Category Three excuse, that is probably a sign you should be forcing yourself to get back in the game somehow, even if you have to do some problem solving and change your routine. Physical activity and movement has a wide spectrum. Even if you have to go on a slow walk instead of your normal powerlifting class, you've overcome your excuse. If you need some inspiration, check out the online media coverage of the Paralympics. These athletes have every opportunity to make excuses for themselves, yet they make none. And neither should you.

View exercise as a privilege, not a punishment

Now that we've established that we aren't going to make any more excuses, we need to step back and take a fresh look at how we think about exercise. I'm willing to bet that many people who loath exercise see it as a punishment of sorts—something they will not and cannot enjoy. But we have to rethink this. The need for intentional exercise is a privilege, not a punishment.

Several years ago, my family spent an entire month exploring the beautiful islands, beaches, mountains, and forests of Ecuador. Despite the many urban areas, Ecuador is considered a developing country with roughly one quarter of its population living in poverty, predominately in the rural areas. When driving through the countryside of Ecuador, it is common to see people tending to crops with hand tools, herding livestock on foot, and carrying the fruits of their labor in baskets on their backs alongside the road. During our travels, we did a lot of walking, moving our luggage, and carrying our small children, but it was difficult to schedule in intentional exercise.

After several weeks, we found ourselves in the tiny, remote town of Cotacachi, where my husband decided to go on a jog one morning. He returned an hour later with a confused look on his face. Seeing him running through the hills of the town in such a leisurely way, with nobody chasing him, the locals had stared at him like he was an alien fresh out of outer space. Some of them even laughed at him. It was then that it occurred to us that many Ecuadorians physically exhaust themselves just to be able to put food on their tables. Seeing a person intentionally physically exerting themselves was a foreign concept to them. And after thinking it through a little more, it did actually feel frivolous.

We had the means to buy anything we really needed or wanted by simply sitting at our computers to earn our living. And the people in this remote area of the world were unable to do any such thing without engaging in difficult physical labor. Later that same year, we traveled to Africa, where we saw people hauling much larger and heavier loads just to provide clean water to their families. This time, we thought it better to do our exercise in a private space—remote hiking trails. If you enjoy food from a grocery store or a local farmer, clean water from a tap or a store-bought bottle, and the ability to earn the money for such commodities without engaging in long hours of back-breaking labor, then your necessity for intentional physical exercise should be viewed as nothing less than a privilege.

Mindset matters

The way you perceive exercise has everything to do with your outcomes. Alia Crum, an associate professor of psychology at Stanford, did a research study in 2007 to better understand the relationship between mindset and exercise-related health outcomes. The experiment involved a group of female hotel attendants. Some of these women were informed that the work they do, which was cleaning hotel rooms, met the surgeon general's recommendations for an active lifestyle. The rest of the women were not provided with this information. The work and behaviors of both groups remained the same throughout the study.

After one month, the group of women who were told that their work was good exercise lost weight, inches from their waists, and body fat, and they experienced improved blood pressures. The uninformed group of women did not experience any of these benefits. This illustrates that the mere *thought* that you are doing something good for your health can build a positive perception of your activity and motivate you to exercise more.

A perhaps more famous study conducted by Alan Richardson in the 1960s also showed how powerful mindset is on sports performance. Participants were divided into three groups meant to measure the effect of mental visualization on basketball free throws. Group one physically practiced free throws for thirty days. Group two mentally visualized successful free throws for thirty days. And group three did neither physical nor mental free throw practice. At the end of the thirty days, group three predictably showed no improvement in free throw performance. However, groups one and two showed an impressive improvement of 24 percent and 23 percent, respectfully. So mental practice through visualization showed nearly the same improvement as physical practice! Apparently there is actual truth to the phrase "if you believe it, you can achieve it."

Mindset can directly affect how you handle challenges, both physical and mental. Researchers who study mental energy and fatigue have discovered that physical fatigue is a highly emotional perception and can therefore be overcome. For those in the back that didn't hear it clearly, *fatigue is a brain-derived emotion, not necessarily a physical limitation.* This means that when we mentally tell ourselves that we can't do something, our physical body follows that advice, even when we are perfectly capable of plowing forward and physically doing that thing.

David Goggins is a decorated US Navy SEAL, an ultra-runner, and a triathlete. He is also an author and public speaker, and he was inducted into the International Sports Hall of Fame. Goggins came up with the popular concept called "the 40 percent rule." The 40 percent rule asserts that we only use 40 percent of our physical capabilities. So as soon as your mind tells you that you're exhausted and unable to go on, you really still have 60 percent left in your tank. Imagine the limitations we mentally impose on ourselves by leaving 60 *percent* of our unrealized potential on the table! There is more interesting stuff about Goggins in Chapter 8.

But one of the reasons why our brains impose such conservative limits on our physical abilities is that the brain frequently works in a teleological way. This means that the brain's thoughts, sensations, and reactions surrounding discomfort all have an important purpose—to protect the body from harm. But we now know that we can train our brains to be much more forgiving when it comes to signals of physical limitations. Nothing truly illustrates this better than static apnea, or underwater breath-holding, while remaining still. At rest, the average person can hold their breath for less than two minutes. That's because our brains have a built-in safety mechanism that stops us from intentionally depriving our bodies of oxygen since we constantly need oxygen to stay alive.

Most experts estimate serious and possibly irreversible brain damage begins occurring after just three to four minutes of oxygen deprivation with death occurring in under ten minutes. Amazingly, a free diver named Aleix Segura Vendrell set a world record in 2016 for a static apnea of 24 minutes and 3.45 seconds. And yes, he is still alive and functioning without brain damage. (I looked it up.) So while it's crucial to take important cues from your mind and body, it is certainly possible to push the limits you *think* you have by teaching your brain that you are capable of successfully pushing farther.

Pushing out of your comfort zone, your brain forms new neural pathways that help you learn and remember that you *can* do challenging things. Over time and with repetition, the stronger these neurons form, the easier the activity becomes. So your brain actually grows and changes to better tolerate tests to your physical limits as you continue to explore them. There is a fitness saying that goes like this: "It doesn't get easier. You just get stronger." And that couldn't be further from the truth both mentally and physically. So wrap your mind(set) around that!

The reward is in the repetition

Repetition is an important key to strengthening your brain and improving your mindset. This is where a lot of people get caught up. People often expect unrealistic results after just a small handful of workouts. They complete six workouts over two weeks and then get discouraged and give up when they don't see the reflection of a lean and muscular build in the mirror. After all, we *are* wired for doing things that produce instant gratification. But while instant gratification can bring us immediate pleasure, it most often comes at the expense of long-term success. And no matter where you're starting from, sustained and improved fitness is always a function of long-term repetition. It is about choosing between what you want now and what you want most. In other words, we should look at the positive effects of exercise as something that will happen gradually with each repetition over a long period of time.

A good analogy for this is how to fill a bucket with water from a slowly dripping faucet. It can be difficult to tell the incremental difference in the water level with each drop, but after many drops over time, the bucket will eventually become full. Each time you work out, you are adding a drop into to your fitness bucket. One workout may yield such unnoticeable results, you could call it a mere drop in the bucket! But many workouts over long periods of time can produce such noticeable results, you might find them overflowing.

A similar analogy exists with saving money for retirement. People who do this successfully put a certain amount of money into a retirement account on a repeat rotating schedule over years and decades. With patience and persistence, they grow a substantial nest egg. Someone seeking instant gratification might put three dollars per day in a savings account for just two weeks and save a whopping forty-two dollars. If they're lucky, that could be enough money to buy a new pair of flip flops. But if they put three dollars per day in a savings account for five years, they will save $5,475, which is nothing to scoff at. In fact, that was close to the amount of money I used as a down payment to purchase my first home back in the early 2000s.

Habits you engage in today and everyday will benefit you years later. In the same way that my saving habits can eventually provide for a comfortable retirement in my old age so will my health and exercise habits. Regular exercise can pay you back with interest by adding healthy, quality years to your life.

Your best cheerleader is you

Speaking of repetition, have you ever noticed the way you talk to yourself in your mind on a daily basis? How do you coax yourself into doing difficult things? What is your internal dialogue if you fail at something, make a mistake, or try something difficult? I will be the first to admit that the topic of positive self-talk is one of my absolute personal weaknesses. Having lived with depression since the age of fifteen, I have strong tendencies toward negative thoughts, feelings, and dialogue about myself. And I know without a shadow of a doubt, that this is the biggest factor preventing me from achieving better health and success in my relationships, business, and fitness.

How do I know this? Because science.

A 2013 study lead by scientist Anthony William Blanchfield tested the effects of motivational self-talk on twenty-four volunteers who were tasked to cycle until exhaustion. Half of the volunteers were given a two-week intensive motivational self-talk program. The other half of the volunteers were not provided with this program. After the two-week program ended, the volunteers were tested again on their cycling times until exhaustion. The group who participated in the motivational self-talk program improved their times to exhaustion by an impressive 18 percent! What's more, the motivational self-talk group reported that their perceived effort was lower, meaning that the intense cycling actually felt easier for them.

What were these magical motivational words? Well, the study participants were instructed to write down positive self-talk statements they had already used in the past and to add other suggested self-talk statements as they saw fit. They chose four favorite motivational statements: two for the beginning of the exercise challenge and two for the end. Then they used these four statements over the two weeks of the study as they practiced cycling and swapped out the ones they felt weren't as motivating in favor of better ones. And that's it! This brings us back to the proof that exercise fatigue is a highly mental and emotional limitation, not a physical one. And it also proves that positive self-talk is one excellent tool we can use to overcome the mental and emotional barriers we impose on ourselves.

Discipline, habits and failure aren't dirty words

Your perception of exercise isn't the only perception that can affect your outcomes. Reframing how you think about discipline, habits, and failure can also have an impact. For me, the term "discipline" used to carry a negative connotation when it came to exercise. I immediately envisioned doing hard things that I didn't want to do over and over again in a painful display of self-torture. But discipline is what helps form habits and forming habits is what makes doing hard things (like exercise) easier. When hard things become easier, you develop more discipline in habitually doing those things. Eventually, this cycle will become something you engage in automatically without having to internally argue with yourself to force the activity.

Think about the things you already do habitually that are so easy you don't even think about them. For me, what comes to mind is putting my seat belt on when I get into the car; it's something I do without a thought. Or driving the same route home from work so many times that I often forget the entire experience even happened once I arrive home. The muscle memory kicks in so strongly there is very little thought involved. How often do you run the steps through your head when you tie your shoes? Sure, at first, I had to use discipline to force myself to do these things until they became habits. But once the habits were formed so deeply they became automatic, something amazing happened: freedom. Discipline becomes freedom when you no longer have to waste precious mental energy on whether or not you are going to do your exercise. The internal mental coaxing, arguing, and forcefulness goes away, which sets you free. Remember all those so-called failures discussed in Chapter 5? What if I told you that the "failures" you've experienced with getting in shape weren't actually failures at all? What if failure only truly exists when you accept it as an endpoint, give up, and stop trying? Failure is only defined by you! But you can redefine it and shift your mindset. We give far too much finality to the word *fail*. We make ourselves believe failure is the end. But we can instead choose to view it as a mere stepping stone toward something better. Failure is a learning opportunity that teaches you what to do next. It doesn't mean you can't do something; it just means you can't do it *yet*. It means that you can try again tomorrow and you might succeed. Failure is not a permanent condition. Nobody can know what they are truly capable of without exploring the edges of their abilities and inviting failure. If you continue to work at something, you may find a new edge.

One of my personal fitness mantras is "if you're not failing, you aren't trying hard enough" because you aren't testing the limits of your abilities. Every time I have described something I've done in my life as a failure, it was because of my own toxic mentality. Deep feelings of frustration, self-pity, and surrender happen to the best of us. It's okay to acknowledge that you are doing hard things. But don't forget to praise yourself for participating in the process—and for your perseverance—even if you aren't pleased with your results at the time. If you get stuck in a rut in which you feel you keep missing the mark, scrape yourself off the pavement and try again and again until you succeed. Athletics and getting or staying fit is a *lifelong* process. It isn't a destination; it's a journey. *There is no finish line.* And as such, you only fail if you give up.

Chapter 7

Get Started

You don't have to see the whole staircase just to take the first step.
—*Martin Luther King Jr.*

Put regular exercise on your priority list. Seriously. Put it right there on top with the other priorities like "pay your bills," "take out the trash," and "buy your groceries." Exercise is important! So make it a priority. If you need to get in shape, lose weight, and improve your health, you *must* make exercise a priority. Kick less important things off your priority list if you have to. And don't make any excuses or concessions. You are going to exercise regularly and you are going to follow through. If you don't prioritize your wellness, you will eventually be forced to prioritize your illness. That is an actual threat from your own body. Tell your employer, tell your family. Once you prioritize exercise, you can work on forming a habit so that it doesn't always feel so forced. We will talk about habit formation in Chapter 9. But until then, make exercise a top priority.

Start slow

In Chapter 3, we talked about the three intensities of physical activity. Recall that light-intensity activities are activities that can be done for the longest duration with the least amount of effort. They can often yield the best results when it comes to losing weight and improving your baseline fitness levels. Remember NEAT—non-exercise activity thermogenesis? This fancy term explains the metabolic benefits gained and the calories burned by the casual activities you do in your life outside of sleeping, eating, and intentional exercise. If your aversion to exercise is severe and/or you feel your weight and fitness levels will make it hard for you to start a more intense exercise routine, start first with increasing your NEAT until you're ready to do more.

Increasing your NEAT is where the rubber meets the road when it comes to the remedy for the sitting epidemic. If your fitness status is in the negative and your weight is very prohibitive to starting more intense exercise, increasing your NEAT is a great place to start. You can easily increase your NEAT and your daily calorie burn by trying just one simple thing.

Don't. Sit. Down.

If you do computer work, get a standing desk. If you are talking on the phone, do it while standing up, or even better, while pacing your home or office. If you typically sit while texting, do it while standing instead. Stand in a waiting room instead of sitting. Stand or pace while waiting for your children at soccer practice. Once you've decreased your sitting time, start doing more! Walk to your mailbox. Shop for your own groceries inside the store while pushing a shopping cart. Wash your car by hand. Increasing NEAT can account for more calories burned than intentional exercise. You'll be amazed at how much of a difference small changes like these can make if you're trying to lose weight. Whether you are ready to sign up for your first 5K run, or you can barely climb stairs, everyone can benefit from increasing their NEAT activities. Modern smart watches and electronic wristbands do a pretty good job of tracking this. For best results, get one that can track your daily standing time, active movements (like folding laundry), and the number of steps you take in a day. At least for the first day, you should do your normal level of activity while wearing the watch to get a good idea of your staring point. Write down where you started and track your progress as a matter of pride and a job well done.

Do something fun!

If you move your body enough with NEAT activity throughout the day, and you're ready to add something more challenging, you've got a really exciting journey ahead of you. This is the part at which we forget the drag of Globo Gyms and remember that exercise comes in so many different, fun, interesting, and exciting forms.

Remember, exercise should not feel like torture, so you'll need to find something you enjoy. My younger self had pigeonholed my mind into the idea that Globo Gyms were the only way to do exercise. What was I thinking? What kinds of things might you have done or wanted to do when you were younger, even if just for fun? My mind draws up rollerblading, bike-riding, trampoline jumping, swimming, soccer, karate, gymnastics, and ice skating. You might not believe this, but you can actually still do most of these things as an adult. Shocking, I know. Or maybe there is something that you have a passion for watching on TV that you've always wanted to try (cough, *American Ninja Warrior*). Or maybe you have a friend that is really into a specific sport, and you think you might want to see what all the hype is about (I'm looking at you, pickleball). If you're like me, you might find more than one activity that appeals to you, which is ideal. A list of, say, five would earn you bonus points. And if you're looking for something obscure, hop online and see what cool and exciting workouts are available in your area. The more you enjoy the activity, the easier it will be for you to adopt it as a long-term habit.

Choose something that favors success

Consider not just how much you might enjoy this activity but also other logistics that might make the activity as easy as possible to carry out. For example, take into account how affordable the activity is, its proximity to your house or workplace, how easily the activity may fit into your schedule, and if this activity is cognitively challenging for you (depending on your personality, this could be a good or a bad thing).

Making your exercise activities as easy as possible to carry out is a huge factor in your success at forming a life-long exercise habit. This might take some retrospective analysis on your part. What some people think will make working out easy could cause quick failures. We all know someone who thought to buy a treadmill or other cardio machine and to put it right in their bedroom in front of the television. For some folks, this is effective, but for many, those machines just become really expensive, ugly furniture. That's because stationary machines can be cognitively challenging. It is worth considering what you have failed at in the past and what inclines you to complete tasks that you find challenging. For example, during college, I learned that it is much easier for me to focus on studying for a test if I go to a quiet place outside of my house with minimal distractions, such as a library. From that experience, I concluded that I would probably not be the type of person who could focus and motivate myself to exercise at home on a regular basis. Consider your personality in relation to the activity you choose and what will help keep you motivated and engaged on a repeated basis.

Research has shown two important factors that help motivate people to adhere to an exercise routine. These are to engage in physical activities that are (1) outdoors and (2) in a group in which, more specifically, you can interact with your co-exercisers. It turns out that vitamin D isn't the only benefit you can get from being outdoors in the fresh air and sunshine. Studies have revealed that outdoor exercise can reduce anger and depression and improve overall mood more than indoor exercise.

. . .

The power of the group

I cannot neglect to give appropriate credence to the power of the group. Group exercise is something I'm passionate about and to which I owe most of my own fitness success. Over the years, some of my group workout partners have described me as competitive. I've always felt misunderstood in this respect, as the term *competitive* can sometimes hold a negative connotation. My biggest competition in every aspect of my life has always been myself. On difficult days, my only aim is to *complete* a workout, no less *compete* in one against anyone else. I'm certainly not trying to *be* the best, rather I'm just trying to *do my* best. I work out with athletes who are better than me for encouragement to push myself to their level, not to prove that I'm better than anyone. Competitive runners use this tactic frequently when they run races with a "pacer." A pacer is a person who runs alongside another runner to help them set personal records. The pacer is not racing the competing athlete; rather, he or she is running to help motivate and guide the racing runner to do his or her personal best. When we can use group exercise in this friendly and motivational way, everyone wins. Humans are, by nature, social creatures. We live in families, we work in teams, and we rely on cooperation amongst ourselves to survive. Exercising in a group has a myriad of benefits. It combats boredom, makes working out more enjoyable, offers built-in accountability, and keeps you motivated. An added bonus is that it enriches your social life. One of the major perks I have always enjoyed about group fitness classes is that the exercises are pre-planned and programmed by someone else on a pre-determined schedule.

All I have to do is show up and do what I'm told to do. The mental stress and energy this has saved me over the years is worth its weight in gold, not to mention providing invaluable guidance. And to be honest, if it weren't for being told to do specific exercises in the company of others who are also doing the same exercises, I would probably never do them at all. For me, group fitness changed my life in a way I can only describe as magical.

Remember Jim Rohn's quote from Chapter 5? "You are the average of the five people you spend the most time with." Well, exercising in a group is the positive influence you've been looking for. A 2010 study in the *Journal of Social Sciences* confirms that people gravitate toward the behaviors of those around them when it comes to fitness and exercise. This means that if you do your exercise with people who are more fit than you, you are likely to work out harder and longer than you would alone or with less fit workout partners. All this is certainly not to say that you should avoid choosing to exercise alone or indoors; it is just highlighting certain factors that might make forming an exercise habit easier and more effective.

Get with a program

With this in mind, if you decide to do your exercise alone, don't reinvent the wheel or go into it without a plan. You want this to be as easy as possible to carry out, so attempting to take on new exercise habits while also carrying the burden of inventing your own training program may work against you. There are a lot of tools at your disposal to help guide you, including a ton of live stream and on-demand workout programs to choose from. Some programs are tied to the use of an actual cardio machine that you must purchase, and some are video series workouts with little-to-no workout equipment required. The variety is endless. Some content is even free. Whatever path you choose, have a solid plan in place in advance and stick to it. If you are starting a cardio routine outside, such as walking, running, or cycling, research tools for beginners for your specific exercise. Even experienced runners use training schedules to train for and complete a marathon or a 5K race, so don't be afraid to really lean into your available resources and dial in on an actual program.

Remember, if you try out a new activity (or even revisit one from your past), and you decide it isn't going to work for you on a long-term basis, you can always try a different activity. When it comes to exercise and fitness, you only truly fail if you give up entirely. So feel free to experiment and fail up, not down! Get out there and be brave enough to be bad at something new.

Set goals

Once you have brainstormed, experimented, and determined what types of activities you enjoy and can realistically incorporate into your lifestyle, you'll need to set some goals for yourself. Setting goals is an important topic. Since you're reading a book about starting and keeping an exercise routine, I'm going to assume this is your overarching goal. Setting a goal to get more exercise on a regular basis, or to get in shape, however, is very broad. As the proverb goes, the only way to eat an elephant is one bite at a time. This couldn't be more true when it comes to fitness. Nobody can get fit from one workout in the same way nobody eats an entire elephant in one dinner sitting.

The biggest favor you can do for yourself when it comes to setting your goals is to reduce them down to smaller, "bite-sized" goals. In my years as a corporate employee, I learned how to set SMART goals for myself in order to achieve career success (and hopefully a pay raise). SMART is an acronym that stands for specific, measurable, achievable, relevant and time-bound. As an example, suppose your doctor recommended that you lose thirty pounds with diet and exercise in order to improve your health markers on your blood laboratory values. If you were starting at a sedentary activity level, a SMART exercise goal would be to walk briskly for three hours each week at a moderate to vigorous intensity (meaning heavy breathing and difficulty having a conversation), for twelve weeks. This type of goal can easily be scheduled out on a calendar with times and dates that can be crossed off your daily or weekly to-do list with a specific, and relatively proximal date at which to celebrate your success.

How you perceive your goals is of utmost importance. If you perceive your goal as narrowly focused, easily manageable, and with proximal success, you are more likely to achieve your goal. Animal and human studies dating back to the 1930s have shown that effort is greatly increased as a finish line or reward is approaching. This means that when you feel you are close to achieving a goal, your motivation improves and you work harder to reach the finish line, a phenomenon called the goal gradient effect. These studies highlight the importance of reducing larger, long-term goals into smaller, more manageable, and less overwhelming goals through which you perceive the finish line as close and within reach. Social psychologist, Emily Balcetis is a published researcher who studies this exact effect in relation to exercise. She ran an experiment with human subjects and tested their running and walking abilities through a course with a visible finish line. When the subjects were asked to narrow their focus on the finish line (as opposed to looking around at their surroundings), the subjects with narrowed focus of attention on the finish line walked or ran 23 percent faster with 17 percent less discomfort. Balcetis's research also shows that people with a narrowed focus of attention to their goal sustained better exercise habits over time.

In other words, you need a concrete plan on how you're going to start your journey and how you're going to reach your goals, in both the long term and short term. If all of this information seems overwhelming (especially if you've been reading or listening to audio and haven't written anything down), don't fret. This book has a companion workbook and planner available, full of specific tools to help guide you into a regular exercise habit. The information about the workbook and planner is provided in Chapter 15. But for now, let's finish learning about how to be successful in forming a fitness routine.

Chapter 8
Remove Barriers and Obstacles

If you find a path with no obstacles, it probably doesn't lead anywhere.
—Frank A. Clark

While we're on the topic of setting goals and creating a plan for success, we must consider all of the potential obstacles that could get in the way. Like everything we set out to achieve in life, progress is hardly linear and often presents challenges that were never anticipated. This is why it is paramount to have a backup plan in place and readiness to solve problems when challenges present themselves.

When I was halfway through my pregnancy with my first son, I was trying desperately to maintain my exercise routine to support healthy weight gain through the end of the pregnancy and to prepare myself for labor and recovery from childbirth. I was regularly attending group exercise classes at a local gym when abruptly and without any warning, the gym owners decided to close their business forever. Feeling fat, tired, and lazy, I could have easily used this as permission from the powers above to just sit on the couch for four months and eat ice cream instead of trying to keep up my regular exercise. But giving up that easily not only felt like I was giving up on myself but also on my unborn child. So I found a different gym with group fitness classes. Although this new gym was not quite as enjoyable, I still went three times per week until I was thirty-eight weeks pregnant. (And I did sit on the couch and eat ice cream a little, too.) When challenges like this present themselves, this is not your cue to give up on meeting your fitness goals. In fact, your ability to solve the problem and plow forward toward your goals will actually strengthen your likelihood for success.

The grit factor

The more often you overcome challenges, the more you will build your capacity for grit, a common characteristic found in successful people. Angela Duckworth, a doctor of psychology known for her research in predicting achievement, found that grit was one of the most important factors in whether a person will achieve success. She defines grit as the tendency to sustain interest in and effort toward very long-term goals. Duckworth studied cadets at West Point Military Academy to try to understand why some cadets dropped out while others finished their military training. She hypothesized that students with stellar high school academic marks, athletic achievement, and high IQ scores would be least likely to drop out. She found instead that grit (as measured by a specific questionnaire) was the common denominator in the successful cadets.

The brain changes and grows in response to challenges when you overcome them. In other words, every time you persevere in the face of adversity, you are teaching your brain that perseverance is possible and rewarding, and that failure is not permanent. One of the most important things you can do to help yourself achieve your fitness goals (and other goals as well), is to overcome barriers, obstacles, and challenges as often as they present themselves. Embrace challenge! For every instance in which you might be tempted to say "I can't because . . . ," make sure you say ". . . but I did anyway" instead. Whining and even cursing is acceptable in my book (literally) as long as you push through the challenge to arrive victorious on the other side. Take every opportunity to prove you are stronger than your excuses and you *will* be.

Use proper tools and equipment

Now that we know we must overcome our obstacles, let's address the list of some common obstacles that can impede anyone's fitness success. First on the list is equipment. The importance of using the proper tools and equipment for any fitness activity you are engaging in cannot be overstated. David Goggins, the Navy SEAL highlighted in Chapter 6 offers a perfect example of equipment challenges in his memoir, *Can't Hurt Me*. Goggins recounts the details of some of the most brutal running and triathlon races imaginable and how he persevered despite having not only a lack of proper training but also a lack of proper equipment for these events.

This man ran a hundred miles in twenty-four hours with only three days' notice, no specific training, and saltine crackers and protein shakes to fuel him.

Later, he completed an Ultraman race during which he swam 6.2 miles, cycled 261.0 miles, and ran 52.4 miles. In this days-long triathlon, Goggins wore an ill-fitting wet suit and rode a bike (including the clip-in shoes) that was fitted to a man much larger than him. He stuffed the shoes with socks and used tape to make them fit better. The result left him with chafed and bleeding arms and severe blisters on his feet. He was also in a bicycle crash that broke his helmet and gave him road rash. He still earned second place in the race, but I can't help but think he would have won first had he used the proper equipment and training tools. Goggins even got the race-day nutrition wrong in both instances with his lack of electrolyte support coupled with his saltine cracker snacks, which should have sent him to the emergency room. If you are brand new to a sport, you don't know what you don't know.

While Goggins is, in my opinion, one of the most amazing athletes on the planet, his experience provides an important lesson for the rest of us: Your performance will only be as good as the tools you are using. Do yourself a favor and perform an internet search to find out what tools you need to succeed in the exercise you're doing. If you are going to begin step aerobics, make sure you wear clothing that doesn't chafe your skin when you move. If you plan to swim laps, make sure you have a comfortable pair of goggles that don't leak. If you are going to take up running, buy proper running shoes that fit you. The wrong footwear was, in part, a big reason I had convinced myself that I could never run a marathon. At face value, these things seem minor, but they can make or break you. Even Olympic athletes experience equipment fumbles, so this is something that happens to everyone. Equipment woes will almost undoubtedly affect you, too, at some point in your journey, and you can overcome them.

Injury and Illness

Speaking of improper equipment, using the wrong stuff is a frequent cause of injury. But even if you are using the proper tools and equipment, you will likely encounter a time when you find yourself nursing an injury or an illness. Obviously, your best bet is to try and prevent injuries or illnesses in the first place, but inevitably one or both will crop up the longer you stick with your exercise habit.

To prevent injury, use the proper equipment, take guidance from those more experienced than you (such as a fellow athlete or a coach), take things slowly at the beginning, and always listen to your body's cues. One of my telltale signs that I am running on shoes that are too worn, is when my knees or hips begin to hurt. Of course, experts recommend that you replace your running shoes every three hundred to five hundred miles, but I'm flawed this way, and I don't bother to count for the sake of my joints. (I'm also a little cheap and try to make the most of running shoes because they are expensive.)

Regardless of how an injury happens, you'll have to be prepared to solve some problems to keep yourself in the game. If you hurt your knee, for example, think of something different you can do that works the other parts of your body while your knee heals. You might start lifting weights for upper body strength, focus on abdominal exercises, or swim laps since swimming is non-weight bearing. Or it may be that the activity you're doing is no longer right for you, and you'll have to switch to a different one permanently. It is very common for runners to retire from running when their joints start to hurt as they age. Often folks opt for less impactful activities, such as cycling or swimming, or they use stationary machines such as an elliptical.

If it is an illness that you are grappling with, take only the time necessary to rest and then ease back into activity as your body allows. If you had a cold and still have a lingering cough, for example, you might switch to some slower walks around your neighborhood, in a park, or at a shopping mall instead of jumping right back into your intense spin classes. It is important to remember that just because you might be hurt or sick does not mean that you should use this as an excuse to stop exercising indefinitely. Being in great physical shape helps your body heal and recover. And persevering through challenges like these will strengthen your body, your mind, and most importantly, your exercise habit.

When it hurts so good

Muscle soreness and broad-scale physical exertion is something that can stop anyone new to fitness in their tracks, and I mean that in a very literal sense. My leg weightlifting days often leave me walking so gingerly, you might easily mistake me for a ninety-nine-year-old woman. Muscle soreness is uncomfortable, but it's a sign you are getting stronger! Drink plenty of water, take over-the-counter pain medications as needed (if your doctor approves), and keep moving to speed up recovery from the soreness.

You will adapt. This adaptation is called hormesis. In biology, the term is used to describe the positive effects of exposing your body to repeated low levels of stress, in this case, exercise. There is, however, a sweet spot with stress exposure as it pertains to exercise. If your workouts yield too much stress exposure to your body, the effect becomes negative, and you risk injury. It is helpful to cycle your workouts with a variety of activities and intensities. For example, if you experience intense muscles soreness from a grueling calisthenics class you are attending twice a week, you could use the days in between to do light cardio to give the sore muscle groups time to recover. Cycling and varying your activities in this way helps to trigger your body's hormetic response, which is what improves your resilience and builds your fitness levels. Again, pay attention to your body's cues. If you find yourself chronically physically exhausted by your exercise routine, it likely means you are doing too much, too frequently.

The schedule and budget dilemma

Legitimate obstacles and barriers to exercise can and will easily morph into excuses if you aren't careful. Two of the most common that I hear when someone is told they need to get more exercise are (1) a lack of time and (2) a lack of money. Without turning this message into unsolicited advice about time management and financial responsibility, I'll try to address both of these barriers.

Time is a finite resource that all of us are stretched across. But if something is important enough, we make time for it. If you can't find at least three open hours in your weekly schedule to dedicate to exercise, then you will have to find something to wipe off the schedule, or something that can be done while simultaneously exercising. For example, if you work remotely and digitally, are there meetings that you can listen in on while walking outside or riding a stationary bike? Or maybe you'll have to give up your weekly watch parties of *The Bachelor*? Or maybe you can arrange a car-pool for your kids to clear up some extra time on your schedule? The demands of managing a household, a family, and a job are no joke. But your ability to juggle these demands will eventually come to a screeching halt if you don't prioritize your health. Talk to your boss, your spouse, and your family members to ask for their support. Hopefully those who care about you most will be willing to help you make your health a priority and clear time in your schedule.

As the saying goes, time is money. If money isn't also your pain point, you can probably pay someone to help you out with tasks that are taking up precious time on that schedule. If money *is* your pain point, like time, this can also be rearranged to prioritize exercise. You may have to trade your monthly shopping mall trip for a gym membership. Or maybe it is as simple as making your coffee and meals at home instead of paying top dollar for someone else to whip them up for you. If there is a will, there is a way. For something that you will actually enjoy doing, and that will help you live your healthiest and longest life possible, you can make it work. Remember that if you don't allocate the time or money for your wellness, you will eventually be forced to allocate both to your illness.

One last pro tip (that gym owners will likely hate me for) on the money front is this: Sometimes monthly memberships are negotiable. There have been times when my husband and I both wanted to join a locally-owned group fitness operation, and instead of paying double (one membership for each of us), we were able to negotiate either sharing one membership between us or buying a second for half price to lessen the pain in the pocket book. I have also done this when signing myself and my children up for sports activities. Many gyms and sports groups have a family discount. It is as simple as a quick ask. The worst possible response is "no" and then you've lost nothing. It may also help to check local deals such as coupons, time-sensitive specials, or contracts between employers and gyms geared toward promoting better health.

Overcoming the ego

The topic of obstacles in fitness will never be complete without addressing egos. First we'll talk about your own, then we'll discuss the egos of others. The *Oxford English Dictionary*'s definition of *ego* is "a person's sense of self-esteem or self-importance." It is related to the idea or opinion you have of yourself; it is your pride. Most of us have feelings of shame or embarrassment about certain aspects of ourselves. As this relates to fitness and exercise, many of us also have shame about our weight, our body shape, and/or our fitness levels.

Having discussed fitness and exercise with hundreds, if not thousands of people, one of the most common pain points I've heard is that people feel they aren't good enough to pursue fitness, or that what they are already pursuing in fitness isn't good enough. I've heard things like "I completed a 5K once, but I walked the whole time so it didn't really count," "I'm too fat to show up to a fitness class—people will laugh at me," or "I'm so out of shape that I will embarrass myself." This kind of mindset prevents people from actually doing better and trying harder for themselves.

Everyone starts somewhere, and many of us fit folks started exactly where you are now. The embarrassment factor can get even more granular when you start to worry about smaller things like "what if I sweat too much?", "what if my hair gets messy?", "what if my body odor is too strong?", "what if I throw up?", or "what if I get out performed . . . by a *girl*?"

I have three words to address all this: Get over yourself. Really.

You are no different than any other human being. We are all imperfect. We all sweat. We all bleed. We all have gross bodily functions. Nobody enjoys eating humble pie, but it is an absolute staple for personal growth. I once loudly broke wind while being physically sat on by a handsome, young college student during a packed jiu jitsu class. (This is a true story.) A lot of people laughed at me. And it was humiliating enough to make me want to quit. But in the end, my best option was to laugh at myself and keep hitting the mats. I am now a purple belt in jiu jitsu. And I definitely wouldn't be telling a story this humiliating without the hope that it would help someone else get over their own fear of embarrassment or at the very least provide a good laugh . . . but I digress. Don't ever let your own feelings of shame or embarrassment get in the way of your success. You are only human, just like the rest of us.

Then there are the egos of others. The ones that perhaps induce feelings of self-consciousness for one reason or another. These are the personalities that radiate intimidation. The athletes who think they are better than you, and they want you to know it. I had the experience of someone in a group exercise class strip weight off of my barbell while I wasn't looking because *they* had decided the weight was too heavy for me. For a time, I often caught the same person monitoring my every move to make sure she always outperformed me. She even shot me dirty looks and verbally put me (and others) down. In short, she was a gym bully and made it a constant point to assert her dominance.

I've run into my fair share of these types of personalities. And what I have gleaned from my interactions with them is that underneath the facade they are outwardly presenting, there is a deep level of insecurity and self-doubt. A vast majority of the time, the way people treat you is a reflection of how they feel about themselves. Do not allow their inner struggles to bleed on you and hold you back from your own goals. Do not be intimidated by people who don't deserve even one second of your attention. You need people who will help you become a better version of yourself, cheer you on, and support you.

The best antidote for an unsavory egotistical gym bully is

to instead model the attitude that you need from others. Cheer people on! Give compliments on their success and encourage anyone who might be struggling. Fitness spaces can sometimes be uninviting, isolating, intimidating, and unforgiving. But they don't have to be if more people can jump on board with the right attitude and influence the community in a more positive direction.

The slip up

Maybe something screwy happened. Maybe your workplace went up in metaphorical flames and you skipped a whole week of workouts playing firefighter. Maybe your spouse and built-in babysitter got sick and the added stress left you skipping the gym. Or maybe you just lost the will. It happens to the best of us. And here's what to do about it: Forgive yourself and start over. It's that simple. Don't call yourself a failure and give up. Don't mentally beat yourself up about it because that will only worsen your motivation to persevere. Just pick up where you left off and move on. It was just a test of your resilience, and you can take the opportunity to pass the test. You will arrive stronger on the other side because of it.

Chapter 9
Make Exercise a Habit

We are what we repeatedly do. Excellence then, is not an act,
but a habit.
—Aristotle

The hardest part about getting in shape and staying in shape is forming a habit of engaging in regular exercise for the rest of your life. If it sounds like a big commitment, that's because it is, which is why many people find it so overwhelming. But the reality is that if you want to enjoy permanent changes to your body, you have to make permanent changes to your lifestyle by forming new habits.

Habits are behaviors we routinely perform on impulse without giving them much thought. A habit is different than a routine in that a routine requires a higher degree of intention and effort. In the beginning phases of forming your exercise habit, you will likely feel uncomfortable because you will need to dedicate the high level of intention and effort required of a routine. But over time, once the routine becomes a habit, you should find it much easier. People often act out of habit, even when it is in conflict with their intentions. Someone may *want* to drink more water, but the habit of drinking the bare minimum already exists as an automatic behavior in their brain circuitry. Therefore, this makes it difficult to adopt a new habit. Our goal is to make exercise a positive habit that we automatically do with little thought attached.

Goal-based and identity-based habits

So what does it actually take to form a permanent habit? Habits are learned behaviors. Experts estimate that between 45 and 70 percent of our daily activities are habitual. Habits can be goal-based or identity-based. Goal-based habits are things you do to achieve something in the short term to illicit a specific outcome. An example of a goal-based habit is training three times per week to complete a hundred-mile cycling race. Goal-based habits are useful when strung together to form an identity-based habit.

Identity-based habits are habits that contribute to an overarching theme to describe who you are. An example of an identity-based habit is riding your bike three times per week to become an avid cyclist. We all know people who formed goal-based habits to lose weight only to gain it all back once the desired outcome was achieved. This is a flaw in focusing solely on an outcome rather than an overarching identity. Someone who wants to lose weight should focus less on being fifty pounds lighter and more on becoming someone who is healthy. To achieve lifelong fitness, we should focus on forming an identity-based habit with a goal of what we want to *become*, not what we want to *achieve*.

Part of what makes this difficult, is that goal-based habits often produce outcomes more quickly, which, when the outcomes are positive, we interpret as rewards—the instant gratification that our brains seek for a dopamine high as discussed in Chapter 4. In contrast, identity-based habits tend to have less time-bound, clearly defined rewards, which makes conjuring and maintaining motivation more difficult. Motivation is largely driven by dopamine and the anticipation of the perceived reward that follows certain behaviors. This is how you can use the goal-setting techniques discussed in Chapter 7 to string goal-based habits together to form a more permanent identity-based habit. The aim is to decide who you want to become and then prove it to yourself through achieving an ongoing series of shorter term, more narrowly focused goals.

Tools for forming habits

But forming a habit is a little more complicated than just setting and reaching goals. To truly form a strong and lasting habit, we need to figure out how to hack into our own brain chemistry a bit further. We know that dopamine is the powerful brain chemical that makes us feel good when we receive a reward for a certain behavior. We can leverage dopamine to induce habit formation because it drives us to repeat behaviors that produce a reward. If that feeling of invigoration and accomplishment that many people feel after they've exercised doesn't feel like enough of a reward, think of other motivating rewards for your work. I happen to enjoy hot showers, so this is always something I can look forward to after my exercise. Additionally, when I've put in thirty to sixty minutes of exercise, my hunger increases, making my meal afterward taste much better. These are things that my brain has come to understand as my rewards for exercise.

Rewards are something that should follow the habit you are trying to perform, but paying attention to the things you do before your habit can also make it easier to carry out. Habit cues, also called linchpin habits are other habits (ideally enjoyable ones) that make a second habit easier to carry out. You can think of linchpin habits as the first link in a chain of reactions, at which one thing leads to another. For example, in my younger years, when I worked a standard eight-to-five, Monday-thru-Friday schedule, one of my favorite parts of my schedule was the habitual clocking out and leaving the office for the day. This linchpin habit was predictable, conveniently determined by my employer, and something I always looked forward to. Unfortunately, for many years, I followed the end of my workday by going home and sitting on the couch to relax. Once I was on the couch, the chance of getting back up, putting on my workout clothes, and going back out to the gym was slim to none. What was worse, the second linchpin habit of going home and sitting on the couch further cued me to mindlessly eat snacks in front of the television. You can see how one thing lead to another, starting with leaving the office.

Once I realized that leaving the office was a linchpin habit promoting my further unhealthy habits, I was able to change how these events were routinely carried out. I decided to pack my gym clothes in the car before work in order to avoid going home after work in the first place, thereby avoiding the lure of sitting on the couch to veg out until it was too late to get to the gym. I harnessed the joy of habitually completing a work day to give me the energy and motivation to head to the gym, and it eventually became a positive cue for my exercise habit. Pharmacists use this technique to help people remember to take their medications. If a medication is to be taken every morning for example, we instruct patients to pair it with a habit they already complete (a linchpin habit) in the morning, such as brushing their teeth or eating breakfast.

By pairing your exercise with positive cues or habits instead of ones that might lead you in an opposite direction, you can train your brain to automatically assign exercise as your next task. When you positively anticipate both the onset and the offset of your habit, you are motivating yourself to complete your habit by triggering the release of dopamine in your brain.

Another tool you can use to increase your likelihood of performing your exercise habit is visualization. Remember the basketball visualization study from Chapter 6? The one in which visualizing successful free throws actually helped people make successful free throws? Well, visualization involves playing the activity in your mind beforehand in detail from start to finish. It works with any type of activity, not just basketball free throws. You can do this by thinking about every step you will take to execute your exercise and what you will gain once it's complete. Do this as much as possible. Make sure, however, that the visualization is a brutally honest account of the difficulty of your activity with a realistic reward. Lying to yourself will actually produce a negative effect on your motivation because visualizing your activity as unrealistically easier and with an impractical reward can set you up for disappointment.

Repetition equals habit strength

With some exceptions, habits generally form through repetition of the activity. When starting a new habit, completing the first series of repetitions will require some discipline and intentional force. With each repetition of the habit, the circuitry of your brain actually changes. Eventually, the habit becomes part of your procedural memory, which helps performing the activity become more automatic and less dependent on goal orientation. In a 2009 study published in the *European Journal of Social Psychology*, scientist Phillippa Lally and her colleagues investigated the process of habit formation in everyday life in ninety-six volunteers. When the (future habit) behavior was performed in a more consistent and repetitive manner, the habit was more easily formed. The researchers found that forming a habit can take anywhere from 18 to 254 days. They considered habits to be well formed or automatic when the participants performed the habit with less mental-activation energy (i.e., the activity didn't feel forced) and the participants completed the behavior at least 85 percent of the time. There is one last important note about this study; missing one opportunity or repetition of the habitual behavior had no effect on the habit formation process. So if you have to skip a workout, don't sweat (literally). Just try not to skip two.

You will know you have formed a very strong exercise habit

when you can still engage in habitual exercise after a change in your environment. For example, if you get a new job, move to a new house, or even move to a new city, and your exercise habit easily continues, you can consider your exercise habit well-formed. I recently moved to a new country with an entirely different landscape, climate, culture, language, and community. To my surprise, the exercise routine that I have carried out in my hometown for the past decade continued despite the drastic change to my environment. Once a habit is well formed, you can and will fight to keep it going no matter the circumstances.

Chapter 10
A Quick Note about Nutrition

Exercise is king. Nutrition is queen. Put them together and you've got a kingdom.
—Jack LaLanne

Exercise goes hand in hand with diet. A quick internet search for "how to lose weight" or "how to be healthier" yields a myriad of advice on both diet and exercise. If you change both your diet and your exercise habits simultaneously, you will almost certainly see much quicker results in your health and body composition.

However, as mentioned in the introduction of this book, my experience as a pharmacist has taught me that making too many drastic changes to your habits and lifestyle at one time increases the likelihood of failure on a long-term scale. This is due to a phenomenon coined "goal competition," which demonstrates that when too many goals are set, they compete for your mental attention. This thereby induces mental fatigue, which in turn, causes motivation to dwindle for one or more of your goals. Of course, you can lose weight faster and see overall changes quicker by changing both diet and exercise habits simultaneously, but those changes are usually short lived and impermanent.

Habits are best formed one at a time to allow for better focus on each habit and enough time to imprint each habit as a permanent fixture in your lifestyle. This is not to say that diet isn't important—it could be argued that diet is actually *more* important than exercise in achieving overall health. It is just to say that changing your dietary habits is better done while focusing on diet alone. So, for the sake of focusing on exercise, this chapter on diet is very brief.

Exercise changes your nutritional needs

Inevitably, as you begin to change your activity levels, your body's nutritional requirements will begin to change. It is important to understand your body's nutritional needs for the activity level you are doing and your overall goals. Without going into great detail for individual circumstances, I recommend doing some internet research and talking to a nutrition expert if you have questions regarding what you need to reach your specific fitness goals for your specific health status. For example, if you want to lose fat and gain muscle, the dietary recommendations can differ greatly between men and women and by age. If you layer any health conditions on top of these specifications, the recommendations may vary even further.

• • •

Balance your energy ins and outs

If you are exercising for weight loss, you'll need a basic understanding of how body weight fluctuates. If you think of your body as a car and the food you eat as the fuel for the car, you can gain a better understanding of how body weight goes up and down. When the car is out of gas, the car can no longer run. Naturally, we need to fill the car with enough gasoline to keep it running. Similarly, our bodies need energy to stay alive and functional. If we filled a car with more gasoline than it could hold, the gas would overflow onto the pavement. But if we fill our bodies with more food (or calories) than it needs for energy, the extra energy overflows into fat storage.

When a person is overweight, this usually means they have regularly taken in more calories (or energy) than they are using for their body to perform daily activities. This is a calories/energy in vs. calories/energy out approach. It is the most simplified explanation for carrying excess weight and does not account for the various hormone imbalances, metabolic diseases, medications, and other health maladies that contribute to carrying excess weight. But in the spirit of keeping this simple, losing weight with exercise means that you must consume the same or lesser amount of energy as you were consuming before you introduced an exercise habit.

This may prove difficult because your body's hunger cues will be stimulated with exercise and you may be tempted to binge-eat McDonald's burgers and potato chips (I might even be speaking from experience). Instead, the best way to control your increase in hunger and provide your body with the proper nutrients is to eat lean protein, good fats, and fibrous, complex carbohydrates to keep you satiated, so you won't eat more than you've burned. This may look like a lightly seasoned, baked chicken breast, a white fish filet, or just some low-fat, low-sugar beef jerky. Veggie sticks with guacamole could work too. I sometimes use low-fat dairy. If you're hungry enough, you will find something you like in these categories even if you haven't gravitated toward it in the past.

What is most important when exercising for weight loss is not putting all (or more) of the calories you just burned through exercise back into your body. Remember that giving your body more energy than it can burn will result in an increase in stored body fat. And similarly, the harder you work and the more you burn energy in your exercise without eating the energy back, the more weight you will lose over time. Even the smallest calorie deficits can induce weight loss. For example, if you are accustomed to eating roughly 2,000 calories daily with a sedentary lifestyle, you could go on short daily walks to burn 120 extra calories, continue eating the same 2,000 calories, and lose one pound per month. If you stepped up your workout intensity, you would lose more weight faster even while keeping your calorie intake the same.

Don't forget the water!

Another cue your body will give you as you increase your activity and fitness levels is thirst. This is caused by an increase in body temperature and loss of water through sweat. Be sure to take your body's cues and drink more water. Ideally, you shouldn't wait to feel thirsty, since thirst is an early sign of dehydration. Dehydration can actually make it harder for you to exercise. It is commonly recommended that you drink water before, during, and after exercise. If you are exercising in a very hot environment or sweat a great deal during your exercise, you may even need to supplement your water intake with electrolytes to prevent cramping. Many sports drinks provide electrolyte support for this reason. Just take note of their caloric value as they often contain sugar as well.

About fitness supplements

As a pharmacist and an athlete, I am asked fairly frequently on my opinion about fitness supplements. It is an enormous industry, with a projected value of over $37 billion by 2027. Like many of the other medications and supplements on the market today, they hold promise for many to be a magic bullet—an easy solution to many physiological challenges pertaining to fitness. Because fitness supplements are not regulated by the US Food and Drug Administration, they are not required to go through scientific studies to prove safety and effectiveness for their advertised purpose.

Fitness supplements promise things like fat loss, muscle growth, improved performance in weightlifting, increased strength and endurance, and quicker recovery. These supplements contain a myriad of ingredients for various purposes, the most common being amino acids, protein, creatine, and caffeine. According to a review of the safety and efficacy of fitness supplement ingredients published by the National Institutes of Health, amino acids, protein, creatine supplements, and other common ingredients in fitness supplements may possibly benefit muscle strength, mass, and response during weightlifting activities, but these studies had limitations and appeared to have the greatest benefit only in elite athletes. Most studies in the review were, at best, inconclusive, and they often had conflicting results.

One of the most common ingredients in fitness supplements, especially those branded as pre-workout supplements, is caffeine. Caffeine reduces perceived pain and exertion and has the potential to enhance performance in endurance type activities when consumed beforehand. There have been a multitude of studies on caffeine and its effects on various processes in the body, including the brain. Most relevant to the fitness discussion, caffeine increases energy, alertness, concentration, and focus. This may come as no surprise to the 94 percent of adults in the US who, in a recent survey performed by SleepFoundation.org, reported regularly drinking caffeine.

You might remember from the study cited in Chapter 7 that people who had a more narrowed focus of attention were significantly more likely to achieve their exercise goals. Caffeine can assist in this way when consumed responsibly. Most people find that consuming between one hundred and four hundred milligrams of caffeine at least three hours (or preferably more) prior to bedtime can produce an energizing and motivating effect to perform a workout and induce the perception that the exercise is easier to complete. Please keep in mind that, like all substances, caffeine may not be the right option for your individual health makeup. Some people find that caffeine exacerbates anxiety, is too dehydrating, or negatively effects their sleep patterns, so you should consult your healthcare professional before adding it to your exercise toolbox.

Everything in life requires a careful weighing of the risks and benefits, so it is important to make these decisions with adequate consideration. With that said, if you decide to use fitness supplements early in your exercise journey, my personal and professional recommendation is to save your money, skip the fancy stuff from the specialty stores, and choose a low-calorie, low-sugar caffeinated beverage from your local grocery store instead. My go-to energy drink is diet soda (save the judgement, please), but I know others who like brand-name energy drinks, black, green, or matcha tea, espresso shots, or just good, old-fashioned coffee.

Chapter 11
Exercise and Women

*A strong woman is a woman determined to do something
others are determined not be done.*
—Marge Piercy

If you happen to have a Y-chromosome in your genetic
makeup, this chapter may seem irrelevant to you. However, if
you are dating or married to a woman, or know any women like
a mother or a sister, you might want to give this chapter a
chance to learn something you don't know. It may even help
you earn some brownie points with the women in your life, or
you might find some of the information also relevant to men. I
don't mean to leave men out, it's just that I'm not a man, and
therefore I'm unable to speak to their experiences. So for the
men in the audience, thanks for holding my purse while I get
this chapter off my chest.

Women are complicated. I only say this because I am one.
We have hormonal cycles and menstrual periods and myriad

concerns about our bodies, our looks, and our social interactions that men couldn't even begin to understand. For this reason, I believe that women's fitness deserves its own chapter.

The wonderland of the female form

Women have a lot of additional considerations that men simply do not have. While everybody sweats, women's body shapes and the tendency for our fitness wear to fit closer to our skin make it a bit different and sometimes more embarrassing. In workout tights and a closely fitted top, crotch sweat, boob sweat, and butt sweat can easily show up as glaring stains during and after an intense workout, and it can even make white fitness wear see-through. Sweat can also completely destroy a carefully done hair and makeup job, leaving you looking worse than if you hadn't bothered doing your hair and makeup in the first place. For women new to fitness, excessive sweat can be a source of concern and humiliation. I only mention it because it's important to know that we all struggle with bodily functions in one way or another that can cause us shame. Knowing that it happens to the best of us may provide some comfort and the ability to simply get over it and stop feeling embarrassed. Indeed sweat (or as I like to call it, "workout glitter") is just one of many details that women worry about when it comes to our bodies during exercise.

Did you know that more than 60 percent of women in our U.S. communities have urinary incontinence? That is according to a study published in 2022 in the journal *Female*

Pelvic Medicine and Reconstructive Surgery. If you're new to the term urinary incontinence, it means we pee in our pants a little. Urinary incontinence can happen when you cough or sneeze, but it can also happen when doing exercises like running, jumping, and weightlifting. It's an extremely common condition, especially among women who have had at least one vaginal birth. So if you find yourself with it, please know that you are not alone. Many women wear special underwear or pads to their workouts, and many more women successfully treat their urinary incontinence by losing weight, getting in better shape, and strengthening their pelvic floor muscles.

Then there are the boobies. Like women themselves, breasts come in all shapes and sizes, and they are all a simultaneous blessing and curse. When I was a teenager, I was lucky enough to be inducted into the Itty Bitty Titty Committee, so I haven't had much of a problem to speak of in the exercise realm (outside of my breastfeeding days). But larger-chested women often find it difficult to do certain exercises if their breast tissue isn't neatly collected into a tightly fitting sports bra. For many women, this is an enormous hurdle into the exercise world, pun intended. Large breasts can really hurt during activities like running and jumping, and it's difficult to find sports bras that can hold everything in while still providing room to breathe. I've known many women who wear two sports bras or even use tape to hold everything in. The good news is that breast tissue is mostly fat, which means that if you are able to successfully lose weight with exercise, you will also likely lose some of that weight in your breasts, making your breast tissue easier to manage for continued workouts. This concept also holds true for belly fat and other fatty tissue. Until you can lose some excess fat, it helps to wear spandex compression or control garments to hold everything in.

Regardless of your size, you are bound to experience chafing in at least one area of your body. This is also a common exercise pitfall for men, but usually in different places on the body. Because women are designed to bear and birth children, women carry more fat than men, and that fat is usually concentrated around the hips and thighs. At the moment of writing this, I am a healthy weight and I consider my body composition to be fairly lean. But every time I run in shorts, my thighs rub together like they are trying to start a fire in a survival situation. When I was overweight, this problem was exponentially worse and also created a barrier to exercise. As an aside, for many women, losing the fat between the thighs to obtain what is called a "thigh gap" is often an impossible feat and an unrealistic beauty standard that can lead to unhealthy eating patterns. But regardless of where on the body it happens, chaffing causes skin breakdown that stings when in contact with your sweat and your shower water in a way that will make you want to grit your teeth and scream.

Again, spandex compression fitness wear has come to my rescue in every possible way. It took me a while to get comfortable in spandex, especially when I was carrying excess weight because spandex can show every curve and crevice. My main contention was that my butt and upper thighs had an embarrassing amount of cellulite that was visible through most leggings. But finally being able to lose the fat was worth it even if my most embarrassing physical flaw was visible. Over the years, fitness wear has come a long way in making garments that smooth out these types of imperfections.

There are also commercial body lubricants meant specifically to reduce chaffing during exercise. These products usually come in a tube or stick that resembles deodorant. Some people have even had success with certain oils such as coconut oil or thicker agents such as petroleum jelly. These items can be a lifesaver for your skin during exercise.

Body image

Certainly cellulite is a common concern for many women, but that doesn't even scratch the surface when it comes to aesthetics. Society has placed a wide variety of pressures and norms on women pertaining to how we should look. I know women who will not leave their house without makeup even if they are going to the gym. As a teenager, I used to wear water-proof mascara to my swim workouts. And what if your hair gets messed up? My best advice for these details is to let them go for the sake of your workout and your health. Regardless of what those fitness models look like on the cover of magazines, most people who are in really good shape do not look like that after their workouts. In fact, in my humble opinion, if your hair and makeup is still in place after your workout, you didn't work hard enough. I always prioritize comfort over fashion when it comes to how I show up for a workout. Maybe I look like a doofus in my high profile foam running shoes, my "I run like the winded" shirt, and my sweat band but I'm happy with my fitness levels, so I care very little.

And then there is the body type stigma. We all have an idea in our heads about what we want our bodies to look like in an ideal world. Again, society has placed this idea in our heads by using media to convince us of what beauty is.

Throw. It. Out.

People come in all shapes and sizes. Only fitness models look like fitness models, and that is why they are fitness models. Remember that you are exercising to be healthy first and foremost, not to be any certain size or shape. A lot of women have asked me if I'm worried about getting bulky from my weightlifting. In the spirit of honesty, it has crossed my mind a time or two. But would I stop because I don't want large biceps? No way! I can out-lift grown men, and people complement me all the time on my arms.

I'm not trying to discourage anyone who has goals to fit into their jeans from college. I'm just trying to impress that there is no perfect body type. Your shape and size will inevitably change many times throughout your life. You should exercise first to be healthy. Positive changes in your body shape and size will eventually arrive and be a welcomed side-effect.

No boys allowed?

When I married my husband (a combat veteran), he told me that he believed women who serve in the military should not be integrated with men in frontline combat (such as infantry). Confused about why he would think this, I asked him to explain further. His reasoning wasn't that women are incapable. (In fact, I've shown him myself how it is possible for a woman to level up to a man in regards to physical fitness and ability). His reasoning was that women would distract the men, therefore creating danger and risk for the entire unit. This threw me for a loop. After a bit of pondering, I understood. There have been times, especially when I was a young, single woman, when working out among men was uncomfortable for me. I felt self-conscious, like a less-than person, and sometimes I felt like I was being watched or judged. As a teenage high school swimmer, I was distracted by a crush I had on a member of the swim team that made it almost intolerable to show up in a swim suit and take my training seriously. I've been part of both female-only and co-ed sports teams and gyms. I now prefer a co-ed workout environment; however, when I was pregnant and post-partum, I would have preferred a female-only gym.

The point here is that you should take some time to consider with whom you would be most comfortable working out with. It's OK to lean into a female-dominant fitness group. I know many mothers who joined baby bootcamp classes after they gave birth and made life-long friends not just for themselves but for their children. Men sometimes have men-only preferences when it comes to certain activities, so women can too.

Ovary-acting

Let's talk about reproductive matters. For women, these can sometimes get in the way of fitness, which is an almost laughable understatement for most of us. Menstrual periods and all of their associated problems can really make it difficult to get off the couch and do life. It's certainly OK to take a menstrual health day. But we women are strong! We can push through anything (even childbirth). So try not to let this become one of your regular excuses for skipping workouts. If you need a day off, reschedule. As long as your healthcare provider approves, take an ibuprofen and get out there! Exercise can help ease menstrual pain and bloating.

Pregnancy is a whole separate animal when it comes to exercise (see what I did there?). Despite what many believe, staying fit and active during pregnancy is actually good for both you and your baby as long as you are healthy and your pregnancy is uncomplicated. Physical activity does not increase your risk of miscarriage, low birth weight, or early delivery. Active women are less likely to experience problems in later pregnancy and during labor. Sticking with a regular exercise routine can ease many of the troubling symptoms of pregnancy. Exercising during pregnancy can also help you cope with and recover from labor and childbirth.

The American College of Obstetricians and Gynecologists (ACOG) recommend pregnant women get at least 150 minutes of moderate-intensity aerobic activity per week, which is the same recommendation the CDC gives to nonpregnant adults. Remember that moderate-intensity means you are breathing through your mouth, you can still talk, but you can't sing. ACOG says that you should pay special attention to your joints, balance, and breathing when exercising during pregnancy because these all change in your body and can make exercise different or more difficult. A hopefully obvious point—pregnant women should avoid contact sports, exercise that creates a risk of falling, exercise that involves extreme changes in altitude, and hot yoga or Pilates. The main message is to listen to your body's cues. If something hurts or is creating extreme discomfort, stop! And always check with your obstetrician before starting any new activity during pregnancy. At your first pregnancy visit, ask to make sure your usual activity is safe and recommended.

But what about after you've had the baby? Well if you had an uncomplicated birth, you can start gentle exercise as soon as you feel up to it. I definitely recommend starting back slowly. Childbirth is very traumatic for many women, both physically and emotionally. And with the added stress of caring for a newborn, coupled with severe sleep deprivation, you'll need to be kind and patient with yourself. Exercise after childbirth helps with recovery, relieves stress, prevents postpartum depression, and helps you lose extra weight you may have gained during pregnancy. It may even help improve the shape of your baby belly. If you had a complicated birth or a C-section, check with your obstetrician to see what they recommend. Again, it is important to listen to your body's cues and take a safety-first approach.

There is a common stigma surrounding mothers and exercise. In the dumpster fire of negativity that is social media, you can find women being shamed left and right for being selfish for spending time to get and stay in shape when they have young children at home (and even while pregnant!). Declines in physical activity in women are heavily associated with the transition to motherhood, especially in working mothers. The balancing act between family and work life often causes women to believe their own health and needs should take a back seat. This cannot be further from the truth. We've all heard the metaphor about the oxygen mask: If you are on an airplane and the cabin loses pressure, put your own oxygen mask on first before helping others. If you aren't doing your best to care for yourself, you will not be able to effectively care for anyone else, including your children. Caring for yourself by allowing time for regular exercise (and hopefully something you enjoy in the process) is not selfish, and mothers should not feel guilty for it. We don't neglect ourselves (or at least we shouldn't) by ceasing to shower or brush our teeth when we become mothers, so why would we do it with exercise? Further, by setting the *example* for your children that exercise and self-care are important for everybody's health, you are setting them up for success in the future. Remember, the study referenced in Chapter 5 showed it is the *mother's influence* that is the strongest and most limiting factor in promoting a healthy lifestyle in children.

Finally there is perimenopause and menopause. Menopause usually happens around the age of 50 when a woman can no longer bear children. The period of time before menopause in which the natural decline of a woman's reproductive hormones begins is known as perimenopause, or menopause transition. This gradual transition can happen years or even up to a decade before menopause fully occurs, typically marked by a woman's last menstrual period. While the idea of menstrual cycles disappearing might seem appealing, perimenopause and menopause come with a whole host of additional problems. On a transient basis, both perimenopause and menopause can cause symptoms such as irregular menstrual bleeding, hot flashes, poor sleep, brain fog, aches and pains, vaginal dryness, recurrent urinary tract infections and more. After these symptoms finally subside, women are often faced with more long-term challenges such as thinning bones, a slower metabolism (which can cause weight gain) and increased risk of heart disease. Like pregnancy, it is imperative for women to maintain an exercise routine throughout perimenopause, menopause and beyond to assist in the best possible health outcomes. The exercise recommendations for perimenopausal women, menopausal woman and postmenopausal women are the same recommendations for all other adults as per the CDC. One thing that should be emphasized is the increased importance of strength and resistance training for the aging body with the goal of preserving lean muscle mass and bone density. These types of exercises promote healthy metabolism and prevent bone thinning—one of the most prevalent health issues in aging women.

Being a woman is no walk in the park. That's why it's so important to be kind to yourself and to other women. Women face enough challenges in life without being hard on one another in the fitness world. Please encourage, inspire, and empower other women! Become the best version of yourself so you can share your best with others. (Girl power!)

Chapter 12

Myth Busting

Do not correct a fool or he will hate you; correct a wise man and he will appreciate you.
—Bruce Lee

The myth that mothers of young children are selfish if they prioritize fitness is only one of the many myths surrounding the fitness industry. There are numerous misconceptions about fitness that lead people in the wrong direction when it comes to their goals. Here I will address seven of the most common myths about exercise.

Myth #1: The myth of spot-reduction

You may have come across folks online or on TV advertising quick workouts to lose belly fat fast or to specifically tone your abs, arms, or butt. They promise things like "in just 15 minutes a day, you can get the six-pack abs you've always dreamed of." I hate to be the bearer of bad news, but these types of workouts with specific body-part-targeted exercises are highly unlikely to deliver their promised results. Spot reduction intended to slim down specific parts of the body is a myth. Currently, there are no robust scientific studies to prove otherwise.

If you want to slim down specific places on your body such as your midsection or your arms, you will need to exercise (and diet) with the intention of lowering your total body fat percentage. In other words, exercise your whole body to lower your overall body fat content instead of attempting to target one specific part of your body. Strengthening specific muscle groups is certainly worth the effort and even recommended, but you won't see much visible difference in the shape or tone of these muscles until you lose the fat surrounding the muscle, which requires you to lose overall body fat. Where your body stores fat and the order in which it is lost are both highly dependent on things like genetics, health status, lifestyle, sex, and age. So unfortunately you don't really get to choose fat reduction for specific areas of your body. But once you lower the fat content from your whole body composition, you will then see your muscle tone that was already existing underneath.

Myth #2: Weightlifting is only for bodybuilders

What if I could recommend an activity for you that would promise a leaner body and a higher metabolism? What if the same activity could also improve your strength, your muscle tone and your bone density? Would you do it? What if that activity involved weightlifting?

Weightlifting can benefit everyone, not just the guy who wants an upper body frame like Mr. Incredible. The medical science available in favor of weightlifting for a healthy body is so strong (pun intended), it is no wonder why the health experts recommends a minimum of two days per week of strength training activities such as weightlifting.

Myth #3: Women shouldn't or don't need to lift weights

I'm not sure where this tomfoolery originated, but this myth has many arms to it. I've heard people say that lifting weights is dangerous for women because women are less physically strong than men. I've also heard women tell other women that lifting weights will make them gain weight and appear "bulky." Whether you are a woman or a man, you might be familiar with the chivalrous act of letting a man do the heavy lifting for a women. While I certainly appreciate and accept the gesture as a woman, this is not an indication that women cannot, or should not, lift heavy objects, especially in an exercise setting.

I once came across an elderly lady in a garden center who needed a heavy bag of soil lifted into her shopping cart. She was standing in the aisle in a helpless fashion, looking at bags of garden soil that were nearly as big as she was. I said to her, "Would you like some help?" And she replied, "No, honey. I'm waiting for a man to come over here and lift this up for me." I smiled. In five seconds flat, I picked up the bag and put it in her shopping cart for her. Shocked at the ease in which I did this, she thanked me and headed to the checkout line. Some people might think physical strength and the ability to lift heavy objects isn't very "lady-like." But for most women, having these traits is not only healthy and empowering, it adds a great deal of utility to many of life's tasks.

And lifting weights for women has all the same health benefits as it does for men. It is no more dangerous than it is for men either, especially when done with the proper form. Further, weightlifting speeds up the body's metabolism to aid in fat loss and will not add muscle bulk to the female form unless done using a carefully calculated program to achieve that specific result. Women generally produce less testosterone than men, a hormone that can promote muscle growth, so for most women it would be extremely difficult to take up weightlifting and accidentally begin resembling Arnold Schwarzenegger. But all this begs the question: Why do so many in our society look down on a muscular female figure? I'll leave you to ponder that one on your own.

Myth #4: The body type myth

This myth can be summed up in one simple phrase: If you don't look fit, you aren't fit. This one really gets my goat. Body type is not an indicator of fitness. Body type is determined by genetics, health status, lifestyle, sex, and age. Because body type is a result of a wide variety of factors, it is different for everyone and can only be controlled to a certain extent. Where someone carries or loses excess weight and their overall shape at different weights is often dependent on factors outside their control. While it is true that most exercise is easier for people who aren't carrying excess weight, just because someone is thin or in a healthy weight range does not also mean they are fit and vice versa. I know many thin people who wouldn't be able to run half a mile or do ten pushups. And I know many people currently carrying excess weight who can outperform most of their peers in a wide variety of fitness activities. Recall from Chapter 1 that regardless of weight, a sedentary lifestyle still increases a person's risk for heart disease, stroke, metabolic syndrome, type 2 diabetes, certain types of cancers, osteoporosis, falls, anxiety, depression, and premature death. So the lesson here is this: Never assume someone's fitness level based on how they look, especially if you don't know them as intimately as you know yourself.

Myth #5: More sweat means a better workout

First of all, I thought we agreed to call it "workout glitter" from now on. All joking aside, the amount of sweat you put out during a workout is a very poor indicator of the benefits of your workout. If you've ever climbed into a car that was parked outside on a hot summer day and immediately started sweating like a sinner in church without any physical exertion, you can understand what I'm talking about. Sweat is just your body's way of cooling itself. Certainly you are more likely to break a sweat during intense physical activity because your body heats up in response to the energy burn. But it is also possible to burn a lot of calories or energy and/or improve strength and condition without breaking a sweat at all, especially with NEAT activities. Even taking a walk in a cold, dry desert environment, for example, may not cause a person to sweat. But this activity could possibly burn more calories than a hot yoga class, after which you may have soaked your shirt. Some people say that "sweat is your fat crying," meaning that sweat is a good indicator your body is burning through its fat stores. As much as I would love this to be true, it isn't.

Myth #6: Morning workouts are better

Now we're starting to major in the minors. Many people prefer morning workouts for a variety of reasons. Motivation levels for exercise tend to be higher after a good night's sleep, and exercise can increase alertness and energy to carry out the rest of the day. But you can benefit from exercise no matter what time of day you complete your workout. There is no scientific evidence that proves certain times of day are better for exercise. So do what is best and easiest for you! You won't catch me doing anything strenuous before the sun comes up, and that works out (literally) just fine for me.

Myth #7: You can eat whatever you want as long as you exercise

Chapter 10 addresses the delicate balance of your body's energy input and output. Whether you are exercising for weight loss or not, giving your body more energy than it can burn will result in an increase in stored body fat. An exception to this is the bodybuilder who is eating a very specific diet to add lean muscle mass, but I promise you these athletes are not eating whatever they want. Since this book is not heavily focused on nutrition, I won't go droning on like a killjoy about the abomination of refined sugar or trans fats, and how you shouldn't eat cake on your birthday (especially because I love cake). But the general scientific consensus is that constantly rewarding yourself for your exercise by eating whatever-you-want foods in whatever-you-want portions is a bad idea and frequently backfires. I'm sorry to say that you can't simply use exercise to erase bad dietary choices.

Chapter 13
Tips and Tricks

Work smarter, not harder
—Allen F. Morgenstern

In 2018, my husband and I took our then six-year-old son to East Africa to climb Mount Kilimanjaro, the highest peak in Africa. During our trek, he set a world record for the youngest climber to summit the mountain unassisted. It was something he really wanted to do, and his father and I wanted to support him. As an overly anxious mother, supporting him in reaching this goal was difficult for me. I worried myself sick, waking up every ninety minutes each night of our trek to make sure my son was still breathing. Even though many years have passed, I still don't know how I managed my fear for his well-being on that mountainside. But I learned a lot of important lessons on Mount Kilimanjaro, and I'll kick off this chapter by sharing two of them with you here.

. . .

The art of distraction

People often asked me "how did you encourage a six-year-old child to complete such a challenging hike?" And here is the answer: We had a lot of momentum to work with in his burning desire to climb the mountain in the first place. But you don't have to be a parent to know that kids are master complainers, and our son is definitely no exception. Whenever he would start to ask about how much longer or how much farther he had to go, that was a cue for me that his mental durability was starting to wane.

So I used one very important tactic: distraction.

I asked him about his favorite things, like his toys, songs, colors, and animals. We played games like Would You Rather or I Spy. I asked him about his dreams. We played word games. We shared stories. And his father and I kept him mentally distracted through each and every one of our mile markers.

This tactic doesn't just work for kids, though. Ironically, I used the same tactic on myself two years later to train for and run my first marathon. A few weeks into my training I found myself falling into negative self-talk during my long runs despite having upbeat music in my headphones. (The sports psychologist recommendation is music between 100 and 150 beats per minute depending on your target intensity, in case you're wondering.) Music just wasn't helping my mind dissociate like I was used to. My brain was tuning it out and defaulting to complaints like "my legs hurt," "I can't finish this," or "I have to walk." So on the recommendation from a friend, I started listening to podcasts instead of music. This did the trick as it kept my mind completely consumed with other things to the point at which I often forgot I was even running. My thoughts were completely diverted from the discomfort I was experiencing and instead were fixated on the content of what I was listening to. I eventually graduated to listening to audio books, which is what lit the spark in me to create the book you are reading (or listening to) right now.

If you are doing exercises that are repetitive and mentally monotonous, especially if you are alone, you can use audio distractions (or video if you're on a stationary machine) to help you get through them. Cardio exercise such as walking, running, or bike riding is perfect for the use of distractions in this way (as long as you remain aware of your surroundings). This is probably the reason why Big Box Gyms strategically place televisions in front of cardio machines. If you find a book or a podcast that you really enjoy, you can even use it as motivation by rewarding yourself with it exclusively during exercise.

The power of the snack

On our son's trek up Mount Kilimanjaro, the only time he shed a tear was on the steepest part of the mountain. We had woken him up at two in the morning to begin the summit. Ice was blowing horizontally, but the climb felt like it was near vertical. We could see the rim of the volcano, the part where the climb leveled out just before the highest point. We had been hiking for at least 5 hours. For the first time during our adventure, he expressed self-doubt. We sat down to rest. And it was then that I realized how low his blood sugar might be. Our guides gave him some juice and chocolate, and in ten minutes time, he was ready to go again. He made it to the summit less than two hours later.

The lesson I learned was this: *Never* underestimate the power of a snack.

Our bodies need energy for activity. If your energy tank is running on empty, your exercise will be a lot harder to complete both mentally and physically. Juice and chocolate were probably not the best choice for our son, but they were our only options at the time, and they gave him the energy he needed to reach his goal. I recommend a small serving of fruit as a pre-workout snack. Fruit provides vitamins, minerals, some hydration, and fiber along with the natural sugars to give your body the energy it needs to crush a workout. If you are training for an activity that lasts longer than an hour or two such as a long hike, a marathon or a triathlon you might even consider some portable energy meant for this type of endurance exercise. Gel packets which are commercially made for this purpose are popular among endurance athletes. Many of these products contain sugar as well as electrolytes, vitamins, minerals and even caffeine.

Laugh it off

I mentioned before that I am an overly anxious mother. More accurately, I'm an overly anxious person in general. I've had anxiety my entire life in connection to just about everything I do—fitness being no exception. Although fitness is one of the best remedies for anxiety, fitness spaces can also sometimes exacerbate it for me, especially in a group setting. If you're like me, just mustering up the courage to walk into a new fitness establishment can be anxiety-inducing enough to deter you entirely. It can feel simultaneously intimidating and isolating.

The best advice I can offer to those who struggle with these social hurdles is not to take any of it too seriously. Exercise is supposed to be fun. I often use humor to squash my anxiety when things get uncomfortable for me. It turns out that our brains' neural pathways are incapable of experiencing humor and anxiety at the same time. Not only does humor and laughing break up discomfort, but it instantly improves your mental state. So break out your fitness joke book and laugh your way through any social discomfort you might run into with your fitness group. Here's one to get you started:

Question: Why isn't the personal trainer paying rent?

Answer: He's squatting (whomp, whomp)

Bonus points if you make anybody, including yourself, smile during a tough workout. Smiling helps the mind dissociate from pain or discomfort the body is feeling.

Don't skip the warm up

If you are opting for moderate-to-high-intensity activities or resistance training, don't forget to warm up and stretch your body before and after your workout. It may sound silly, and if you're like me, you may be tempted to skip out on this step (I sometimes do when I'm short on time), but warming up and stretching your muscles is actually really important. Warming up increases your body and muscle temperature, which improves blood and oxygen flow. Better blood flow will make it easier for you to get the most out of your workout. The warmup and stretching process also helps improve your muscle and joint elasticity and flexibility, which will help reduce your risk for injury.

Tips for weight loss and fat loss

How do you exercise to specifically achieve fat loss and weight loss? The first rule of thumb is that more movement is better. The more you can move your body in any possible way throughout the day, the better. The second rule is to mix your workouts up between high-intensity interval training (HIIT) and strength or resistance training that targets the whole body. These types of workouts are the most effective at burning body fat.

Boot camp-style workouts, circuit training, and cross training activities are good examples of HIIT. HIIT workouts focus on quick bursts of hard, mouth-breathing exercise with rest time in between sets. HIIT is the type of exercise where "less is more." The focus is on expending more energy within smaller time frames (usually fifteen to twenty minutes), but the calorie burn actually continues hours after the workout is completed. These types of workouts are extremely effective and great for people who are trying to lose weight, but are short on time.

Strength and resistance training to build muscle can play a major factor in shedding excess fat. This is why weightlifting and other types of strength training can be so life-changing for people carrying excess weight. Increasing your body's muscle mass helps you burn more calories at rest, meaning an increase in metabolism. Let me reiterate that. More muscle mass means you will burn more calories when you are lying in bed or sitting on the couch. Muscles super-charge your body's engine to make it burn more calories, more quickly. So make sure to incorporate muscle building exercises into your routine if your goal is to lose excess weight.

The last important rule to follow when exercising for weight loss and fat loss is to operate on a calorie deficiency. This means that you will need to consume less caloric energy (food and caloric beverages) than you burn on a daily or weekly basis. Regardless of how you achieve this, more exercise will prove immensely helpful.

When to rest

By now you might be asking "If more movement is better, then when should I rest?" If you are new to exercise, you will need to start out slow. In the beginning, you will feel more tired and experience more muscle soreness than you are used to. You may need to rest every other day at first. Over time, as your body condition improves, you should be able to do more and fill in those rest days with lower intensity exercises such as walking, gentle water aerobics, or yoga. It's important to keep moving, especially when you're sore or tired. Take these opportunities to prove to yourself you can do it even when things get hard. Remember that the brain changes and grows in response to challenges when you overcome them. Overcoming challenges helps to rewire your brain and increase your overall momentum to continue your habit.

. . .

Make exercise as easy as possible by reducing the mental load

Forming new habits can be a challenge, so we want to tap into every possible way to make forming an exercise habit as easy as possible. Chapter 7 impressed upon the importance of finding an activity that you enjoy and is not overly difficult for you to carry out. Both of these factors will not only lesson the mental energy it takes to perform your habit but help to keep you motivated to repeat it over and over. Preserving mental energy is a very important point. If you are too rigid with your exercise routine, you might actually be working against yourself by creating too heavy of a mental load. When something causes you a great deal of mental stress, your physical capabilities can actually diminish.

A recent study led by Walter Staiano and published in the *International Journal of Sports Physiology and Performance* highlighted just this. Sixteen men and women were subjected to mentally demanding tasks for ninety minutes before being asked to lift weights. They were then asked about their perceived levels of exertion. The results showed that when the subjects were mentally fatigued, they felt higher levels of exertion during physical exercise. Other studies have revealed similar findings. This shows how critically important it is to preserve mental energy in order to succeed in carrying out physical activity. It also highlights the reason why many people succeed at doing their exercise in the morning after a good night's rest and before the brain gets a chance to exert itself with the daily grind.

Besides staying away from too much rigidity in your exercise routine, there are other things that can help lessen your mental load and make it easier for you to get your exercise done. Have you ever tried to manually push a broken-down car? It is much harder to get the car moving from a standstill than it is to *keep* it moving once the wheels are already rolling. The same is true with people! The hardest part of doing tasks that you perceive as challenging is to start. Starting difficult tasks requires what is called activation energy, or the brain energy it takes to set yourself in motion. Remember that our brains are wired to take the path of least resistance. This means that we should take steps before the scheduled task in order to set ourselves up for success. We can do this by removing any time and effort barriers in advance of our scheduled exercise.

For example, if you are going on a bike ride, you can check some things the night before: (1) Make sure your bike is mechanically ready with wheels on the ground, (2) your water bottle is filled and on the bike, (3) your clothes, shoes, and helmet are set out in advance, and (4) your route is mapped. By doing these things, you have not only saved yourself time later but removed the physical and, more importantly, the mental loads required of you in order to start your workout. Your goal is to make it as easy as possible when it's time to get started, therefore drastically decreasing the amount of activation energy you will need. Packing your gym bag in advance or keeping your gear in your car are some ideas. Some people set their workout clothes out the night before their workouts or even sleep in them!

A commonly cited study on the topic of exercise and habit formation is "Combining Motivational and Volitional Interventions to Promote Exercise Participation: Protection

Motivation Theory and Implementation Intentions," published in 2002 in the *British Journal of Health Psychology*. It's quite the academic mouthful of jargon, but I'll break it down into a few sentences. The study used 248 participants, separated into three groups, to see what types of things could increase a person's likelihood of building better exercise habits over a two-week period. The results revealed one thing that could increase the likelihood of carrying out exercise by nearly threefold. What was it? A written plan for the following week that stated when (specific day and time) and where (specific place) their exercise was to be completed. This is one of the important reasons why this book has an accompanying workbook and planner that can be purchased on the website. It will hopefully be another useful tool to help you achieve fitness success.

Why does this work? Because it takes the mental energy expenditure away from the moment of activation. By preplanning an activity, you won't need to spend time or energy thinking about how, when, or where the activity will happen—or even if you are going to do it—when the time comes to start the activity. Steve Jobs famously did this with his clothing choices by wearing the exact same outfit every day: a black turtleneck, blue jeans, and New Balance sneakers. Since his outfit was already preplanned, Jobs knew that he would save the mental time and energy he would have needed to choose his clothing every morning for other, more important decisions. In his later years, Albert Einstein did the same thing with his wardrobe.

. . .

The power of you

My pharmacy practice has taught me that, as the saying goes, you can lead a horse to water, but you can't make him drink. I have shared helpful information, advice, and instructions with thousands of people about how and why to take medications and improve their health. And I was often faced with the disappointing reality that, like God, I could only help those who help themselves.

So I will end this chapter with one final thought: You can read the books and buy the fitness equipment and pay for the memberships and even work through the workbook, but those things will go to waste without your consistent attention to and use of them. There is no magic bullet or potion to set you in motion toward fitness other than your own true volition. *You* are the sole person in charge of your health, your fitness, and your life. *You* are who allows others to influence you in positive or negative ways. *You* are the only one in the driver's seat traveling your fitness journey. So strap in, start that engine, and put your foot on the gas. You've got this.

Chapter 14

The Story of My Personal Fitness Journey

Every experience in your life is being orchestrated to teach you something you need to know to move forward.
—Brian Tracy

Exercise never came easy to me and I never considered myself naturally athletic. I was raised by a struggling single mother who set a good example for me by prioritizing regular exercise and supporting any sports activities that piqued my interests. I was able to try a wide variety of activities throughout my life, most of which I wasn't very good at. I spent many years doing trial-and-error exercise habits and activities. The things I enjoyed the most, I honed and developed my skills for. I've lost and gained the same ten to thirty pounds many times since puberty. I've suffered my whole life with anxiety, depression, and a whole host of other health issues, several of which I previously used, unfortunately, as excuses for why I wasn't in better physical shape. During my many years as a full-time pharmacist, I saw firsthand every consequence of poor diet and lack of exercise up to and including death. But there was one life-shattering event that made me see my health and my able body from an entirely different perspective.

Charlie was my most present and consistent father figure. He frequently stepped in when I needed help with something. He loved me even when I was a bratty teenager and didn't deserve it. He was a New Yorker, an avid cyclist, a photographer, and a good person.

In 2005, when I was finishing college, Charlie started noticing that his feet were dragging. Several years later he could barely walk. My heart broke when he couldn't walk me down the aisle at my wedding in 2009. He was later diagnosed with amyotrophic lateral sclerosis (ALS), also known as Lou Gehrig's disease. ALS is a progressive neurological disease that causes muscle weakness and gradual degeneration of the vital functioning of the body, eventually leading to death. His last years of life were spent confined to an armchair, unable to move most of his body. In the end, he could hardly speak or eat, and he couldn't move any of the muscles of his neck, causing his head to hang down onto his chest like a rag doll when we propped him upright. My mom and I took care of him until he passed away in the summer of 2011. He was fifty five years old.

Seeing Charlie's gradual decline and eventual inability to move had a very profound impact on me. I started to become much more aware of my body's abilities. When I stood up to walk, even to my kitchen or to use the restroom, I felt thankful for my working legs. I started running more, swimming more, cycling more. I did a five-mile open-water swim, a triathlon, and some 5K running races. I took up kickboxing and Brazilian jiujitsu. The year Charlie died, I joined a CrossFit gym. Aside from the obvious physical and mental health benefits of exercise, I had found a much deeper purpose for it. I began to set and chase fitness goals the same way I did with personal and professional goals. I racked up enough fitness achievements to fill a resume of sorts—something I could look back on with pride and fulfillment in case I was ever permanently bedridden.

This wasn't the first nor the last time tragedy struck during my lifetime. Almost everyone experiences tragedy and misfortune at some point in their lives. In these moments, it is easy to fall victim to feelings of profound sadness, hopelessness, and grief and slip into habits that can negatively effect your health. But I believe victimhood is self-defined. It is our ability to learn and respond positively and resiliently to tragedy and misfortune that helps us make life's lemons into lemonade.

I don't do these physical activities to impress anyone. I don't do them to look good in a bathing suit. I don't do them to compete or win trophies. My body is healthy and *alive* and *able*. So I *use* it and *care* for it, and I feel so much gratitude for every day that I can move.

The opportunity for fitness is a privilege that isn't afforded to everyone. Please don't take your body for granted. If you have working arms and legs, *use them*. Some people don't.

Caitlyn Tanner, Pharm.D

And someday you might not be able to. If you can use your muscles and exercise your body, you should. Exercise is the best way to show gratitude to your body and your physical capabilities. It's part of being fully alive.

Chapter 15
Recap and Conclusion

There is an epidemic of sedentary behavior in the developed world. We simply do not move our bodies enough or engage in regular exercise routines, which is making us collectively sick. Regardless of body weight and composition, exercise is one of the best remedies for a wide variety of maladies. Physical fitness is one of the best ways to prevent costly medical interventions, and it is proven to extend both the quality and quantity of your life. Despite this common knowledge, regular exercise is a habit that many people find extremely difficult to adopt for a variety of reasons. In order to overcome these difficulties, we must hack into our brain chemistry, change the way we view exercise, and take detailed steps to develop a strong, effective, and enjoyable exercise habit. Starting slowly and prioritizing more movement throughout our daily lives is paramount. Forming new habits and overcoming obstacles can be challenging, so use every tool at your disposal to improve your chances of success. Everyone is different, so find what works best for you and lean into it.

Ten key points to remember:

1. Find exercise activities you enjoy, and you will find it easier to prioritize them.

2. Taking part in group exercise and/or outdoor exercise with people more fit than you has been shown to improve your likelihood of completing your exercise on a regular basis and improve your fitness levels.

3. Consider potential ways to make it easier for you to exercise, such as making it convenient relative to your work schedule or commute and preplanning your workouts.

4. Use goals to guide behaviors by making short-term, narrowly focused goals with a visible finish line and stringing these together to reach long-term goals.

5. Use repetition and overcoming challenges to rewire your brain in order to form a strong exercise habit.

6. In order to lose weight with exercise, you must move more and eat less, with the goal of operating in a calorie deficit, working toward some regular, intense, mouth-breathing workouts, and building muscle mass.

7. Drinking enough water, eating a light snack, and getting enough sleep helps your body prepare for increased physical activities.

8. Preplanning your workouts with a specific date, time, and activity will increase your likelihood of performing exercise.

9. The hardest part of forming new habits is starting, and the best time to start is now.

10. You are the only one who has the power to change your habits and your life.

Getting fit and staying in shape may have proven to be difficult for you in the past, but as long as you have the will, you can walk the path toward success. Basic human abilities can be grown. Your journey might get tough, but you're tougher. You *can* do difficult things, and they will make you better each time you try *even if* the result isn't always your definition of a perfect success. It is better to try and fall short than to never try at all. And it is better to keep trying than to give up on yourself. Your improved health will reward you beyond your expectations, and you deserve the reward. Physical fitness does not measure intelligence. It does not measure kindness. It does not measure creativity. It does not measure a great many of other characteristics that make a person valuable to the world. But it does measure your ability to love yourself enough to prove it.

The Exercise Hack Workbook and Planner

You can find *The Exercise Hack Workbook and Planner* on the website www.theexercisehack.com. The workbook portion will help guide you step by step to get you started on your fitness journey, and the planner will help keep you accountable and motivated. The website also includes the scientific information and studies referenced in this book, free bonus material, fun fitness merchandise, and other tools and recommended reading.

If you choose to share your fitness journey on social media, consider using the hashtag #theexercisehack to inspire others and let the fitness community cheer you on!

Thanks so much for reading!
Can I please ask a small favor?

It's hard to believe, but I spent almost two years writing this book! It also took courage to share publicly such personal stories and some of my greatest flaws and vulnerabilities. I really hope you liked the book and found it helpful, interesting and motivating. It would mean a lot to me if you could leave a review using the link below. My deepest gratitude for your support.

SCAN TO REVIEW

REFERENCES

Ainsworth, Barbara E., William Haskell, Arthur S. Leon, David R. Jacobs Jr,
Henry J. Montoye, James F. Sallis, and Ralph S. Paffenbarger Jr. 1993.
"Compendium of Physical Activities: classification of energy costs of
human physical activities." *Medicine & Science in Sports & Exercise* 25,
no. 1 (January 1993): 71–80. https://doi.org/10.1249/00005768-
199301000-00011

American Academy of Dermatology Association. 2021. "How your workout can
affect your skin." Last updated May 27, 2021. (n.d.).
https://www.aad.org/public/everyday-care/skin-care-
secrets/routine/workout-affect-skin

American College of Obstetricians and Gynecologists (ACOG). 2022.
"Exercise During Pregnancy." Last updated March 2022.
https://www.acog.org/womens-health/faqs/exercise-during-pregnancy.

American Heart Association – Eastern States. 2018. "National Cycling Day."
May 14, 2018. https://easternstates.heart.org/national-cycling-day/

Bajić, Senka, Dragoljub Veljović, and Borko Đ. Bulajić. 2023. "Impact of
Physical Fitness on Emergency Response: A Case Study of Factors That
Influence Individual Responses to Emergencies among University
Students." *Healthcare* 11, no. 14 (July 19, 2023): 2061.
https://doi.org/10.3390/healthcare11142061

Balcetis, Emily, Corey Guenther, Joshua Pesantes, and Shana Cole. 2021.
"Where You Look and How Far You Go: The Relationship Between
Attentional Styles and Running Performance." *Current Research in
Ecological and Social Psychology* 2 (2021): 100014.
https://doi.org/10.1016/j.cresp.2021.100014.

Balcetis, Emily, Matthew T. Riccio, Dustin T. Duncan, and Shauna Cole. 2019.
"Keeping the Goal in Sight: Testing the Influence of Narrowed Visual
Attention on Physical Activity." *Personality and Social Psychology Bulletin*
46, no. 3 (July 19, 2019): 485–496.
https://doi.org/10.1177/0146167219861438.

Basso, Julia C. and Wendy A. Suzuki. 2017. "The Effects of Acute Exercise on
Mood, Cognition, Neurophysiology, and Neurochemical Pathways: A

REFERENCES

Review." *Brain Plasticity* 2, no. 2 (March 28, 2017): 127–152.
https://doi.org/10.3233/BPL-160040

Begot, Isis, Thatiana Peixoto, Laion R. A. Gonzaga, Douglas Bolzan, Valeria D. W. Papa, Antonio C. C. Carvalho, Ross Arena, Walter J. Gomes, and Solange Guizilini. 2015. "A Home-Based Walking Program Improves Erectile Dysfunction in Men With an Acute Myocardial Infarction." *The American Journal of Cardiology* 115, no. 5 (March 2015): 571–575. https://doi.org/10.1016/j.amjcard.2014.12.007

Blanchfield, Anthony William, James Hardy, Helma Majella De Morree, Walter Staiano, and Samuele Marcora. 2014. "Talking yourself out of exhaustion: the effects of self-talk on endurance performance." *Medical Science Sports Exercise* 46, no. 5 (2014): 998–1007. doiDOI: 10.1249/MSS.0000000000000184. PMID: 24121242.

Boere, Katherine, Kelsey Lloyd, Gordon Binsted, and Olave E. Krigolson. 2023. "Exercising Is Good for the Brain but Exercising Outside Is Potentially Better." *Scientific Reports* 13, no. 1 (2023): 1–8. https://doi.org/10.1038/s41598-022-26093-2.

Burke, Shauna M., Albert V. Carron, Mark. A. Eys, Nikos Ntoumanis, and Paul A. Estabrooks. 2006. "Group Versus Individual Approach? A Meta-Analysis of the Effectiveness of Interventions to Promote Physical Activity." *Sport & Exercise Psychology Review* 2, no. 1 (February 2006): 13–29. https://doi.org/10.53841/bpssepr.2006.2.1.13.

Canadian Broadcasting Corporation (CBC). 2018. "Humans have not evolved to exercise, says Harvard prof." *CBC Radio* (2018, February 23). Last updated February 9, 2011.
https://www.cbc.ca/radio/thecurrent/the-current-for-feb-9-2021-1.5906730/humans-have-not-evolved-to-exercise-says- harvard-prof-1.5907580 #:~:text= It%20turns%20out%2 C%20that's%20an, Do%20Is%20Healthy%20and%20 Rewarding.

Centers for Disease Control and Prevention. 2022. "CDC Releases Updated Maps of America's High Levels of Inactivity." Last modified January 20, 2022. https://www.cdc.gov/media/releases/2022/p0120-inactivity-map.html

Centers for Disease Control and Prevention. 2022a. "Childhood obesity facts." Last updated May 17, 2022. https://www.cdc.-gov/obesity/data/childhood.html

Centers for Disease Control and Prevention. 2022b. "How much physical activity do adults need?" *Move More; Sit Less*. Centers for Disease Control and Prevention. https://www.cdc.gov/physicalactivity/basics/adults/ index.htm#:~ :text=Adults%20should%20move%20more %20and,activity%20- gain%20some% 20health%20benefits.on.

Centers for Disease Control and Prevention. 2022c. "Obesity is a Common, Serious, and Costly Disease." Accessed July 20, 2022. Centers for Disease Control and Prevention. https://www.cdc.gov/obesity/data/adult.html

Centers for Disease Control and Prevention. 2023. "Benefits of Physical Activity." Centers for Disease Control and Prevention, Accessed August 1, 2023. https://www.cdc.gov/physicalactivity/basics/pa-health/index.htm

Cheema, Amar and Rajesh Bagchi. 2011. "The Effect of Goal Visualization on Goal Pursuit: Implications for Consumers and Managers." *Journal of Marketing* 75, no. 2 (March 2011): 109–123. https://doi.org/10.1509/jmkg.75.2.109.

Cheval, Boris, Eda Tipura, Nicolas Burra, Jaromil Frossard, Julien Chanal, Dan Orsholits, Rémi Radel, Matthieu P. Boisgontier. 2018. "Avoiding sedentary behaviors requires more cortical resources than avoiding physical activity: An EEG study." *Neuropsychologia* 119 (October 2018): 68–80. https://doi.org/10.1016/j.neuropsychologia.2018.07.029

Citadel Faculty and Staff. 2018. "Citadel-led study reveals threat to U.S. military readiness due to unfit recruits," *The Citadel Today*, last modified January 11, 2018. https://today.citadel.edu/citadel-led-study-reveals- threat-to-u-s-military-readiness-due-to-unfit-recruits/

Citadel Faculty and Staff. 2019. "U.S. Army aims for tougher fitness standards despite amount of overweight recruits," *The Citadel Today*, last modified January 1, 2019. https://today.citadel.edu/army-fitness-citadel-study- recruits-obese/

Cole, Shauna and Emily Balcetis. 2021. "Motivated Perception for Self- Regulation: How Visual Experience Serves and Is Served by Goals." *Advances in Experimental Social Psychology* 64 (2021): 129–186. https://doi.org/10.1016/bs.aesp.2021.04.003.

Collins, Tim. 2018. "Humans are hardwired for laziness because evolution favours conserving energy." *Mail Online*, September 19, 2018. https://www.dailymail.co.uk/sciencetech/article-6184411/Humans- hardwired-laziness-evolution-favours-conserving-energy.html

Colman, Andrew M. 2009. "Pleasure principle." *A Dictionary of Psychology*

REFERENCES

(3rd Edition). Oxford: Oxford University Press.
https://doi.org/10.1093/oi/authority. 20110803100331556

Crum, Alia J. and Ellen J. Langer. 2007. "Mind-set matters: exercise and the placebo effect." *Psychological Science* 18, no. 2 (February 2007):165–71. https://doi.org/10.1111/j.1467-9280.2007.01867.x10.1111/j.1467-9280.2007.01867.x. PMID: 17425538.

Duckworth, A. L., C. Peterson, M. D. Matthews, and D. R. Kelly. 2007. "Grit: Perseverance and Passion for Long-Term Goals." *Journal of Personality and Social Psychology* 92, no. 6 (2007): 1087–1101. https://doi.org/10.1037/0022-3514.92.6.1087.

Duckworth, Angela and James J. Gross. 2014. "Self-Control and Grit: Related but Separable Determinants of Success." *Current Directions in Psychological Science* 23, no. 5 (2014): 319. https://doi.org/10.1177/0963721414541462.

Elsevier. 2022. "Obesity threatens U.S. military readiness, experts say." *ScienceDaily* (May 6, 2022). www.sciencedaily.com/releases/2022/05/220506102623.htm

Graupensperger, Scott, Jinger S. Gottschall, Alex J. Benson, Mark Eys, Bryce Hastings, M. Phil, and M. Blair Evans. 2019. "Perceptions of Groupness During Fitness Classes Positively Predict Recalled Perceptions of Exertion, Enjoyment, and Affective Valence: An Intensive Longitudinal Investigation." *Sport, Exercise, and Performance Psychology* 8, no. 3 (2019): 290. https://doi.org/10.1037/spy0000157.

Hagura, Nobuhiro, Patrick Haggard, and Jörn Diedrichsen. 2017. "Perceptual decisions are biased by the cost to act." *ELife* 6 (February 21, 2017). https://doi.org/10.7554/elife.18422

Herlambang, Mega B., Niels A. Taatgen, and Fokie Cnossen. 2021. "Modeling Motivation Using Goal Competition in Mental Fatigue Studies." *Journal of Mathematical Psychology* 102 (2021): 102540. https://doi.org/10.1016/j.jmp.2021.102540.

Hull, C. L. 1934. "The Rat's Speed-of-Locomotion Gradient in the Approach to Food." *Journal of Comparative Psychology* 17, no. 3 (June 1934): 393–422. https://doi.org/10.1037/h0071299.

Kemp, S. 2022. *Digital 2022: Global Overview Report.* DataReportal (May 4, 2022). https://datareportal.com/reports/ digital-2022-global-overview-report

Kemp, S. 2022a. *Digital 2022: Time Spent Using Connected Tech Continues to Rise*. DataReportal (May 4, 2022). https://datareportal.com/reports/digital-2022-time-spent-with-connected-tech

Kivetz, Ran, Oleg Urminsky, and Yuhuang Zheng. 2006. "The Goal-Gradient Hypothesis Resurrected: Purchase Acceleration, Illusionary Goal Progress, and Customer Retention." *Journal of Marketing Research* 43, no. 1 (February 2006): 39–58. https://doi.org/10.1509/jmkr.43.1.39.

Knapik, J. J. 2015. "The Importance of Physical Fitness for Injury Prevention: Part 1." *Journal of Special Operations Medicine* 15, no. 1 (Spring 2015): 123–127. https://doi.org/10.55460/as9h-fo5o

Koster, Olinka. 2007. "Fit? Half of us can't even touch our toes," DailyMail.com (September 28, 2007). https://www.dailymail.co.uk/health/article-483782/Fit-Half-touch-toes.html

Lacharité-Lemieux, Marianne, Jean-Pierre Brunelle, and Isabelle J. Dionne. 2015. "Adherence to Exercise and Affective Responses: Comparison Between Outdoor and Indoor Training." *Menopause* 22, no. 7 (July 2015): 731–740. https://doi.org/10.1097/GME.0000000000000366.

Lally, Phillippa, Cornelia H. M. van Jaarsveld, Henry W. W. Potts, and Jane Wardle. 2010. "How Are Habits Formed: Modelling Habit Formation in the Real World." *European Journal of Social Psychology* 40, no. 6 (2010): 998–1009. https://doi.org/10.1002/ejsp.674.

Li, Norman P., Lynn K. L. Tan, and Brian K. C. Choy. 2021. "Evolution, Biology, and Attraction." *Oxford Research Encyclopedia of Psychology* (June 28, 2021). https://doi.org/10.1093/ acrefore/9780190236557.013.302

Limbers, Christine A., Christina McCollum, Kelly R Ylitalo, and Mikki Hebl. 2020. "Physical Activity in Working Mothers: Running Low Impacts Quality of Life." *Women's Health* 16 (2020). https://doi.org/10.1177/1745506520929165.

Locke, Edwin. A. and Gary P. Latham. 1985. "The Application of Goal Setting to Sports." *Journal of Sport Psychology* 7, no. 3 (September 1985): 205–222. https://doi.org/10.1123/jsp.7.3.205.

Lopez, Nanette Virginia, Mark H. C. Lai, Chih-Hsiang Yang, Genevieve Fridlund Dunton, and Britni Ryan Belcher. 2022. "Associations of Maternal and Paternal Parenting Practices With Children's Fruit and Vegetable Intake and Physical Activity: Preliminary Findings From an Ecological Momentary Study." *JMIR Formative Research* 6, no. 8 (August). https://doi.org/10.2196/38326

McLellan, Tom M., John A. Caldwell, and Harris R. Lieberman. 2016. "A Review of Caffeine's Effects on Cognitive, Physical and Occupational

REFERENCES

Performance." *Neuroscience & Biobehavioral Reviews* 71 (2016): 294–312. https://doi.org/10.1016/j.neubiorev.2016.09.001.

Mendes, Márcio de Almeida, Inácio da Silva, Virgílio Ramires, Felipe Reichert, Rafaela Martins, Rodrigo Ferreira, and Elaine Tomasi. 2018. "Metabolic equivalent of task (METs) thresholds as an indicator of physical activity intensity." *PLOS ONE* 13, no 7 (July 19, 2018). https://doi.org/10.1371/journal.pone.0200701

Milne, Sarah, Sheina Orbell, Paschal Sheeran. 2002. "Combining Motivational and Volitional Interventions to Promote Exercise Participation: Protection Motivation Theory and Implementation Intentions." *British Journal of Health Psychology* 7, no. 2 (May 2002): 163–184. https://doi.org/10.1348/135910702169420.

National Center for Chronic Disease Prevention and Health Promotion (NCCDPHP). 1997. "Guidelines Guidelines for forwSchool and Community Programs to Promote Lifelong Physical Activity Among Young People." *Journal of School Health* 67, no. 6 (August 1997): 202–219. https://doi.org/10.1111/j.1746-1561.1997.tb06307.x

National Heart, Lung, and Blood Institute. 2022. "Physical Activity and Your Hearth: Types." Last updated March 24, 2022. https://www. nhlbi.nih.gov/health/heart/physical-activity/types#:~:text= The%20three%20main%20types% 20of,heart%20and%20lungs%20the%20most

National Institute on Aging. 2024. "Four Types of Exercise and Physical Activity." National Institute on Aging. Accessed on April 14, 2024. https://www.nia.nih.gov/health/exercise-and-physical-activity/four-types-exercise-and-physical-activity

National Institutes of Health, Office of Dietary Supplements. 2024."Dietary Supplements for Exercise and Athletic Performance." Last updated April 1, 2024. https: //ods.od.nih.gov/factsheets/ ExerciseAndAthleticPerformance-HealthProfessional/.

Noakes, Timothy David. 2012. "Fatigue Is a Brain-Derived Emotion That Regulates the Exercise Behavior to Ensure the Protection of Whole Body Homeostasis." *Frontiers in Physiology* 3 (2012). https://doi.org/10.3389/fphys.2012.00082.

Patel, Ushma J., Amy L. Godecker, Dobie L. Giles, and Heidi W. Brown. 2022. "Updated Prevalence of Urinary Incontinence in Women: 2015–2018 National Population-Based Survey Data." *Female Pelvic Medicine & Reconstructive Surgery* 28, no. 4 (January 12, 2022): 181–187.

https://doi.org/10.1097/spv.0000000000001127.

Plante, Thomas G., Meghan Madden, Sonia Mann, Grace Lee, Allison Hardesty, Nick Gable, Allison Terry, and Greg Kaplow. 2010. "Effects of Perceived Fitness Level of Exercise Partner on Intensity of Exertion." *Journal of Social Sciences* 6, no. 1 (January 1, 2010): 50–54. https://doi.org/10.3844/jssp.2010.50.54.

Police, Sara B. and Nicole Ruppert. 2022. "The US Military's Battle With Obesity.," *Journal of Nutrition Education and Behavior* 54, no. 5 (May 2022): 475–480. https://doi.org/10.1016/j.jneb.2021.12.003

Qiu, Yan, Benjamin Fernández-García, H. Immo Lehmann, Guoping Li, Guido Kroemer, Carlos López-Otín, and Junjie Xiao. 2023. "Exercise sustains the hallmarks of health.," *Journal of Sport and Health Science* 12, no. 1 (January 2023): 8–35. https://doi.org/10.1016/j.jshs.2022.10.003

Richardson, Alan. (1967). "Mental practice: A review and discussion: II." *Research Quarterly,* 3838, no. 2: 263–273.

Ryosuke, Oizumi., Sugimoto Yoshie, S., and& Aibara Hiromi, A. (2021). "The association between activity levels and skin moisturising function in adults." *Dermatology Reports* 13, no. 1 (March 17, 2021). https://doi.org/10.4081/dr.2021.8811

Sandoiu, Ana. 2019. "Adult obesity: Is childhood sugar intake in the '70s to blame?" *Medical News Today* (2019, September 25, 2019). https://www.medicalnewstoday.com/articles/326449

Staiano, Walter, Lluis Raimon Salazar Bonet, Marco Romagnoli, and Christopher Ring. 2023. "Mental Fatigue: The Cost of Cognitive Loading on Weight Lifting, Resistance Training, and Cycling Performance." *International Journal of Sports Physiology and Performance* 18, no. 5 (May 1, 2023): 465–473. https://doi.org/10.1123/ijspp.2022-0356.

Stohl, Emma. 2023. "Childhood Obesity in the United States." *Ballard Brief.* (August 31, 2023). https://ballardbrief.byu.edu/issue-briefs/childhood-obesity-in-the-united-states

Temple, Norman. J. 2022. "The Origins of the Obesity Epidemic in the USA–Lessons for Today." *Nutrients* 14, no. 20 (October 2022). https://doi.org/10.3390/nu14204253

Thompson Coon, J., K. Boddy, K. Stein, R. Whear, J. Barton, and M. H. Depledge. 2011. "Does Participating in Physical Activity in Outdoor Natural Environments Have a Greater Effect on Physical and Mental Wellbeing than Physical Activity Indoors? A Systematic Review." *Environmental Science & Technology* 45, no. 5 (2011): 1761–1772.

REFERENCES

https://doi.org/10.1021/es102947t.J.

Warburton, Darren E. R., Crystal Whitney Nicol, C. W., and Shannon S. D. Bredin. 2006. , S. D. (2006). "Health benefits of physical activity: The evidence." *CMAJ : Canadian Medical Association Journal* 174, no. 6 (March 14, 2006): 801--809. https://doi.org/10.1503/cmaj.051351

Wood, Wendy and Dennis Rünger. 2016. "Psychology of Habit." *Annual Review of Psychology* 67 (2016): 289–314. https://doi.org/10.1146/annurev-psych-122414-033417.

Yang, Pei-Yu. Y., Ka-Hua Ho, K. H., Hsi-Chung Chen, H. C., &and Meng-Yueh Chien, M. Y. 2012. "Exercise training improves sleep quality in middle-aged and older adults with sleep problems: a systematic review." *Journal of Physiotherapy* 58, no. 3 (September 2012): 157–163. https://doi.org/10.1016/s1836-9553(12)70106-6

About the Author

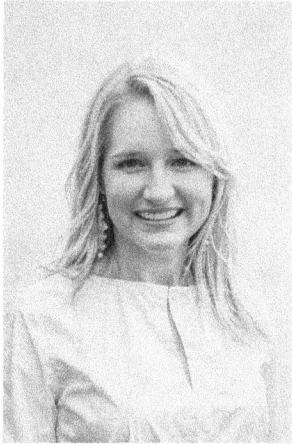

Caitlyn Tanner is a pharmacist, athlete, entrepreneur, science enthusiast, wife and mother of two. After nearly two decades of practice in the medical field helping treat chronic illness, she developed a passion for disease prevention through promoting healthy habits and lifestyle changes. Having experienced her own health issues and challenges with forming healthy habits, she sought to connect with people in an authentic, candid and practical way through her writing. With this book she hopes to help and inspire people to take control of their health. When she isn't testing the limits of her abilities with things like swimming Alcatraz, climbing Mount Kilimanjaro or practicing her hand-stand walk, you can find her outside on a leisurely jog with her running partner, the family dog. Learn more about Caitlyn and her other work at www.theexercisehack.com

www.ingramcontent.com/pod-product-compliance
Lightning Source LLC
Chambersburg PA
CBHW070807280326
41934CB00012B/3088